'I KNOW WHO CAUSED COVID-19'

'I KNOW WHO CAUSED COVID-19'

PANDEMICS
AND XENOPHOBIA

ZHOU XUN AND **SANDER L. GILMAN**

REAKTION BOOKS

Published by
REAKTION BOOKS LTD
Unit 32, Waterside
44–48 Wharf Road
London N1 7UX, UK
www.reaktionbooks.co.uk

First published 2021
Copyright © Zhou Xun and Sander L. Gilman 2021

Printed and bound in Great Britain
by Bell & Bain, Glasgow

A catalogue record for this book is available from the British Library

ISBN 978 1 78914 507 6

CONTENTS

PREFACE:
IN TIMES OF STRESS

The title of this book should be a parody, yet it is not. Carol Midgley in *The Times* of London set the tone in April 2020: 'Although I obviously believe the one that it was Greta Thunberg who caused Covid-19 to reverse climate change and that Russia has released lions to enforce social distancing. Although I also believe that the dinosaurs helped to build the pyramids and I have been quite tired lately . . .'.[1] We have all been tired recently, not only by COVID-19 but by the incessant and often crude attempts to deal with the emotional impact of the pandemic. Fear leads not only to denial ('it's all a hoax') but to quackery ('Hydroxychloroquine is an easy cure') and accusations of conspiracy ('Bill Gates/George Soros/the Communist Party of China planned this and it came out of their labs'). Yet these claims also have everyday real-world impacts. At the end of 2020 a bomb planted by Anthony Quinn Warner in downtown Nashville which destroyed city blocks was seemingly intended to demolish an AT&T transmission building, because the bomber believed that the new 5G network caused COVID-19. Dr Simone Gold, one of the loudest advocates for hydroxychloroquine, a quack cure for the virus advocated by Donald Trump (along with injecting bleach), was one of the insurrectionists who invaded the U.S. Capitol on 6 January 2021, where she filmed herself in the Rotunda decrying the new vaccine as an 'experimental, biological agent deceptively named a vaccine'.[2] 'I know who caused COVID-19,' they all screamed, as 'they were given power over a fourth of the earth to kill by sword, famine, and plague, and by the wild beasts of the earth death and destruction followed them', if we may cite the Book of Revelations (6:8). Our book looks at how accusations of all sorts about causing or transmitting or controlling the pandemic created communities, many of them online and thus global, but all of them intended to deal with the anxiety inherent in such a global pandemic. Fear has consequences, for individuals and for communities.

THUS OUR book was written, rewritten and rethought at the height of the 2020 COVID-19 pandemic. It concludes with a view back towards early twentieth-century pandemics, but begins in December 2019 with the initial appearance of a novel coronavirus, now identified as the severe acute respiratory syndrome coronavirus (2 SARS-COV-2), the cause of the disease later named COVID-19. Our timeline ends on 20 January 2021 with the inauguration of Joseph Biden as the president of the United States, in the midst of a catastrophic and deadly pandemic and a flawed rollout of the first vaccines made available – virtually a year to the day after the first case of COVID-19 was identified in the country. We have updated our findings as much as possible from our closing date to the date when our book went to press in April 2021. This is an arbitrary moment, but seems a necessary one to provide an arc to our narrative about blame and retribution.

The book thus examines a topic to which both authors have contributed essays and books over the decades. It is, one can say, a coming to terms with a lifetime of pandemics and epidemics, each of which was in the moment unique, never before experienced, staggeringly appalling in the threats to life and the functioning of society: from HIV/AIDS in the 1980s, which continues to cost tens of thousands of lives annually, to the various patterns of infectious disease – bovine spongiform encephalopathy (mad cow disease), foot-and-mouth disease, SARS, MERS, Zika – that have dominated the mass media as well as state public health authorities over the decades, to finding ourselves locked down in Washington and Essex, lecturing and living remotely, along with much of the world. Again, we might add, what became evident for both of us over the course of 2020 is that one of the common threads in our experience of disease as historians is that there was and is a substantial psychological component, both to the individual and collective processing of the fear generated by the disease and to our social responses to the stresses generated. What we are trying to do in this book is to examine how the complexity of such ways of dealing with fear mirror as well as distort what one can label our 'normal' manner of ego defence. There is nothing inherently pathological in the mechanisms that Anna Freud outlined in her *The Ego and Mechanisms of Defence* (1936). The defences of the ego under normal circumstances can take the form of repression, displacement, denial, projection, reaction formation, intellectualization, rationalization, undoing and sublimation as well as identification with the aggressor or self-hatred. What are of interest in this present book are not the underlying substrata but rather the rhetorical and thus political functions that these mechanisms manifest. How do we articulate repression, denial, identification and so on in very specific settings and circumstances – explicitly, in these cases, those generated by the experience of living in cultural communities in the time of COVID-19? We have approached this question as sceptics, knowing full well that as we too live in the shadow of this experience, our readings are always fragmentary and unfinished. We rely for our materials, as can be evident, on the mass media, print and virtual, as well as on the critical literature. The latter has been expanding over the experience of the pandemic and we see in it also a reaction (as we understand our own work to be) to this experience.

1

XENOPHOBIA AND COVID-19

In times of stress such as during epidemics, ancient prejudices and primeval fear, always beneath the surface, can be
brought to life to haunt us. When recounting the tale of the
Plague of Athens in 430 BCE, the historian Thucydides blamed
the Ethiopians for causing the epidemic, which led to the moral
disorder that took hold of the city and had long-lasting negative
consequences.[1] From this first account of a pandemic in the
West, the fear of the Other has become a permanent feature
of all epidemics.[2] Counter-epidemic hysteria always attributes
new diseases and their mutations to the actions and behaviours,
malevolent or merely different, of the Other. Unfamiliar cultural
practices, anything 'foreign', from foods to body odours to the
colour of the skin, as well as patterns of sociability, are defined
as threats that covertly or overtly undermine *our* health and the
fabric of *our* perfect/normal society. Thus the identity of a group
is often constituted, not solely by common interests, geography
or even politics, but by a clear definition of where danger lies. In
our age of growing anxiety over globalization and migration as
well as excessive lifestyle, the fear of the diseased stranger and
infectious contact as well as 'horrors of diversity and excess'
are replicated and proliferated at an alarming rate through viral
media, and have become equally contagious and dangerous.[3]
The now common metaphor of the virus for exploding online
communication, a virtual viral infection, reflects our underlying

fears. Viruses and the fear they generate are just information badly processed. Normally they sit inert, sometimes for thousands of years. Indeed, we live in a web of viruses, fungi, prions and bacteria. Human networks bring them to life and transmit them to others. What Thucydides did in his relatively cheap and easily copied papyrus scrolls is now replicated a billion times over on the World Wide Web.

SOCIAL PSYCHOLOGY has long recognized this need to project anxiety and has given it a label: xenophobia.[4] Its older roots, as one of the authors of this essay has argued, lie in the debate in the Enlightenment about whether a misperception of difference that leads to antipathy is a normal or a pathological response.[5] Are we pre-programmed to so respond to perceived difference or is this a learned experience? By the early twentieth century this debate remained unresolved. In English, according to the *Oxford English Dictionary*, the word first appeared in 1909 in the *Athenaeum*: 'Those whose sense of justice and fair play is not impaired by prejudice or "xenophoby".'[6] Not too much later Sigmund Freud, for example, sees this as a natural process for the collective. For, as he noted in his 1921 paper on mass psychology, 'We are no longer astonished that greater differences should lead to an almost insuperable repugnance, such as the Gallic people feel for the German, the Aryan for the Semite, and the white races for the coloured.'[7] For Freud this is an inherent problem to be overcome, but the irrationality of the fear of the Other is not 'unnatural'. Is xenophobia a problem that defines individual or collective belief and action? Is it an aberration or a natural phenomenon?

With pandemics/epidemics, as we are seeing with COVID-19, to no one's surprise, familiar social and ethnic out-groups have been the target of this seemingly irrational xenophobia. All the appointed culpable groups are visible within the cultures in which they live and, indeed, beyond them. Individual members of these groups, often easily identifiable by appearance or dress, have been accused of transmitting the disease and attacked on the street. Yet, as with its murky origin, one of the most pernicious aspects of covid-19 is that it seems to be spread as much (if not more) by asymptomatic as it is by symptomatic individuals.[8] The anthropologist Mary Douglas noted decades ago that

> fear of danger tends to strengthen the lines of division in a community. If that is so, the response to a major crisis digs more deeply the cleavages that have been there all the time. This will mean that if there is a big inequality of wealth, the poor will suffer more than if the distribution were more equitable. If there is violent xenophobia, the foreigners will be blamed and pogrommed more.[9]

Out-groups, so defined by Mary Douglas in the age of HIV/AIDS, today have become stigmatized as innocent targets of the anxiety and anger of those labelled as at risk of the disease and thus the implied cause of its transmission. There is a clear consensus today that such xenophobia is morally wrong and inappropriate in a civil society, that these charges point to a false morality, for a pandemic terrifies the moralist, as its cause is always someone else's sin:

> During this so-unwelcome, unanticipated period of social distancing, protective masks, and lockdowns, the temptation to act out against others seen as responsible for our annoyances and aggravations can be almost overwhelming.

But should we succumb to it, whatever biases we might already have held against our (imagined) enemies – whether because of their race, religion, or ethnicity – can eventuate in victim-inspired, but nonetheless culpable, behaviors. In times of elevated stress, even subtle, dimly recognized prejudices can be blown out of all proportion, compelling us to react in unprecedented ways.[10]

Rather than being judged as individuals, people are seen as members of a collective and are targeted for something over which they have little or no control. Older models of group stigmatization are simply brought to life as a means of psychological and social herd immunity in limiting and locating the observer's valid if inchoate fears. We would not argue with these general statements.

But what do we do when the charge is verifiable? What do we do when the charge is cast in terms that promote obfuscation? How do we deal with the onerous and difficult question of mixing or working through obnoxious stereotyping with actual fact-finding? What happens when history is indeed put to the task of explaining, but instead masks and distorts? When what is called a category error, made by lumping all individuals or communities into an overarching constructed classification, be it labelled 'race', 'ethnicity', 'class' or 'gender', turns out to be flawed in the generalization, but more or less correct in any particular case?[11] When the hoary claim that stereotypes contain a 'kernel of truth' suddenly seems to be accurate? How can we examine causation along with the analysis of stigma without falling into the trap of seeing all categories as constructed and then read as fictive?[12] What happens when victims are simultaneously perpetrators? How do we analyse their responses and be aware of the heightened atmosphere and its history that shape them? As the medical anthropologist David Napier has noted, commenting on a petition concerning the pandemic circulated by the United Nations Secretary-General António Guterres, "'We're all in this together" rings hollow when so many feel we are not.'[13]

When we look at xenophobic discourse towards populations as well as individuals in those populations, to use the standard term of art from public health authorities, we might first consider how we define a population. The role of public health at the very beginning of the twentieth century was seen as 'the science and art of preventing disease, prolonging life, and promoting health through organized efforts and informed choices of society, organizations, public and private, communities, and individuals'.[14] Note that the term 'population' has not yet entered the field. The word is taken from statistics and means merely the set of objects selected as linked by one or more common features.[15] Today we speak of population health, which looks at 'the health outcomes of a group of individuals, including the distribution of such outcomes within the group'.[16] It is comprised of three main components: health outcomes, health determinants and policies.[17] To this, one can add the age of mass media and global access to information and misinformation, and the question of how one understands and processes such components.[18] Such a definition, while functional, is often at odds with the sense of what such a designation means in practice, as the seeming scientific neutrality of these terms is experienced and understood in very different ways by those impacted.

Let us rather layer these meanings masked by the term 'populations' with those associated with that of 'community', a concept that also appears in the early twentieth-century definition of public health and has recently been used over and over again in the discussions of COVID-19. Here the political theorist Benedict

Anderson is helpful. In his widely cited *Imagined Communities: Reflections on the Origin and Spread of Nationalism* (1983), he argues that communities as such arise when the national state becomes so large or so diffuse that a symbolic register – the flag, leader, language, race or, indeed, health and illness – come to be the focus of the newly constituted symbolic community.[19] Anderson's now classic formulation holds that the very concept of the nation arose in the Enlightenment at the moment when there were no longer uniform symbolic networks, such as the divine right of kings, to define the national community. The symbolic nature of such new communities must seem as 'natural' as did the older systems. Anderson writes,

> in everything 'natural' there is always something unchosen. In this way, nation-ness is assimilated to skin-colour, gender, parentage, and birth-era – all those things one cannot help. And in these 'natural ties' one senses what one might call 'the beauty of *gemeinschaft*.' To put it another way, precisely because such ties are not chosen, they have about them a halo of disinterestedness.[20]

Here the symbolic overlay of the idea of population health (or illness) becomes yet one more 'disinterested factor', which is, on the contrary, a highly invested manner of defining the community. This is a symbolic rethinking of John Rawls's notion of 'social unions' in his *Theory of Justice* (1971), in which individuals complete themselves by joining or constituting such communities, for good or ill. A population is not a community; a community is not a population.

Like Anderson, William Bloom stressed that 'national identity . . . is that paradigm condition in which a mass of people have made the same identification with the national symbols – have internalized the symbols of the nation – so that they may act as one psychological group when there is a threat to, or the possibility of the enhancement of, these symbols of national identity.'[21] But Bloom also recognizes that as much as we identify with certain symbols, we also define ourselves against other symbolic registers, as we are 'in a state of permanent competition with its international environment'.[22] Here Bloom makes it clear that he is writing about the constitution not only of the nation-state but of the very idea of a community in the post-Enlightenment era. Such nation-states incorporated into themselves other communities, sometimes forcefully. In doing so they denied that there could ever be a 'multicultural nation', a nation that had a dominant symbolic register but was simultaneously able to allow conflicting symbolic communities to exist within its bounds. Enlightenment thinkers such as J. G. Herder, in his *Ideas for a Philosophy of the History of Mankind* (1784–91), rejected the very idea of a multilingual, multicultural nation that could incorporate competing symbolic vocabularies, thus enabling a citizen to shift codes. (He really didn't like Switzerland!)[23] Yet the lived reality is that a citizen can and does shift codes from within to without any given community identity. One can belong to different, sometimes conflicting communities simultaneously, but such code switching is always fraught with perils.

When an individual or a group is confronted with such inherent contradictions, when two symbolic systems defining identity clash, or seem to clash, the resulting double bind, as Gregory Bateson noted more than half a century ago, seeks alternative explanations. These then resolve the 'paradoxes' that result when 'two or more messages – metamessages in relation to each other – . . . [generate] a confusion of message and metamessage' by providing a contingent answer that seems to resolve the paradox, but simply masks it.[24] When being blamed morphs into placing blame, it is important to understand such a process as being one of boundary-building within a symbolic (imagined) community. It is the identification with the collective, no matter how contradictory the responses or how heterogenous such a collective actually is, that is at the centre of this process. It is a flight into the symbolic realm rather than an act of rational choice.[25]

Sigmund Freud's understanding of the wellspring of mass psychology and its construction of difference through the drawing of symbolic boundaries can also be of help. In his 1921 essay *Group Psychology and the Analysis of the Ego*, he began with the claim that had long been established in the psychological literature of the late nineteenth century concerning collective behaviour that 'a group is extraordinarily credulous and open to influence, it has no critical faculty, and the improbable does not exist for it.' But what he adds is that collectives 'think in images, which call one another up by association (just as they arise with individuals in states of free imagination), and whose agreement with reality is never checked by any reasonable agency'.[26] These images are the core of the symbolic vocabulary that both Anderson and Bloom gesture towards. Hatred is at the core of such images but its wellspring is fear. 'A group impresses the individual as being an unlimited power and an insurmountable peril. For the moment it replaces the whole of human society, which is the wielder of authority, whose punishments the individual fears, and for whose sake he has submitted to so many inhibitions.'[27] What motivates the collective is a fear that now has a clearly definable source. That such fear comes to be what Jacques Lacan, following Claude Lévi-Strauss, labels the symbolic register, that 'aspect of experience whereby signification is introduced as distinct from representation. Representation requires resemblance, whereas signification rests on difference: At its most basic level it rests on the absence of the object named, on the difference between word and thing, and on the differences among words.'[28] It is difference that generates the images of health and illness, of stranger and familiar, of cause and effect. The symbols of difference, simultaneously imaginary, symbolic and real, imbricate actual human beings. They form our relationship with those living in our world, seen as existing in and through a world of images.

One response to living in this world of comparison and contrast is to call up known symbols of defining oneself within the community and in times of COVID-19. As we shall discuss in much more detail in Chapter Five, one of the favoured responses is to evoke 'freedom', both as an individual and as a collective. Freedom becomes a litmus test of whether actions intended to control the pandemic are defined as unacceptable to the collective. In the Western tradition, from the Greeks on, individual autonomy was recognized as having inherent boundaries within the social fabric, what Freud described as constituting the superego that internalizes these limitations of the ego. They can be so fully internalized that they become habit and therefore are naturalized; we do not think of them as external limits on action and behaviour but simply as part of who we are, such as those taboos that forbid incest, as Sigmund Freud observes in *Civilization and Its Discontents* (1930).[29] Indeed, Lévi-Strauss, in *Elementary Structures of Kinship* (1949), uses the term 'symbolic register' as well as the example of incest, seeing the incest taboo as a mandate to marry beyond the kinship group.[30] All these mandates seem natural to those who are bound by them. But if we become consciously aware of them through their integration into our symbolic world as a negative image, we sense a sudden limitation on our autonomy, on our freedom. Mask-wearing in the West would seem to be neutral – indeed, invisible – in that sense, but once it became a political issue, we became aware of it as a symbol and it came to be an ideological statement, for good or ill. In Asian countries, such as Japan, Thailand or South Korea, where mask-wearing was commonplace before the pandemic as a sign of polite recognition of the possibility of placing one's compatriots at risk, no such limitation on freedom was perceived.[31] In Hong Kong, during the SARS pandemic in 2003, pro-democracy lawmakers campaigned for everyone to wear a mask as a form of resistance to the Hong Kong government invoking the old British colonial quarantine rules. Such radical rules were criticized by different social groups in Hong Kong as infringements on individual civil liberties.[32] In the liberal West too, social distancing or distancing socially became favoured by many, as it was seen as a more humane alternative to what were understood early on as draconian quarantine practices, which had literally disappeared from contemporary medical and political vocabularies until the present pandemic.[33]

When symbolic images pointing the finger at a community as responsible for plague morphs into that community in turn placing blame on yet another collective, it is important to understand this as reinforcing boundaries for that symbolic (imagined) community. Not we, they imagine, but those ones over there are the ones at fault – the outsiders, the Jews, the government, the mask-wearers. But it is the identification with a collective through this symbolic vocabulary, not an individual's response, that is vital. It is each member of a community that uses such images to define themselves within the social herd, no matter how contradictory the responses or how heterogenous such a collective actually is. It is a flight into the symbolic realm rather than an act of rational choice. Thus many other approaches that define risk in terms of individual action seem also to be less effective in explaining why and how blame is laid. Daniel Kahneman and Amos Tversky's work on 'incorrect' perspective in making choices may be at play when different ways of judging/dealing with the same risk are presented to the audience at large.[34] They reported in 1979 on an experiment in which one group of undergraduates was asked to imagine the rates of death from a range of causes from cancer to homicide. Another group was asked simply to guess the difference in rate between the undefined categories of 'natural' as opposed to 'unnatural' causes. This latter group scored the potential for a natural death radically lower than for an unnatural one, underestimating the probabilities for natural causes and overestimating those for unnatural causes. Kahneman and Tversky noted that 'probability judgments are attached not to events but to descriptions of events . . . the judged probability of an event depends on the explicitness of its description.'[35] The reality is that 'unnatural' causes were and are part of a highly charged discussion in the public sphere in the United States at the time (about minorities, crime, gun control, punishment), while 'natural' causes, including potentially infectious diseases, were not an active part of the public sphere. Indeed, some of the diseases, such as cancer, were in the 1970s actually socially taboo topics.[36]

Likewise, Kahneman, in his justly praised notion of 'fast thinking', argues that such rapid individual responses to external stimuli distort decision-making, causing what seem to be intuitive responses to known situations to simply be wrong.[37] But we do this not as individuals but through our collective values as members of a community that defines difference in ways that seem unreflected because of the community's collectively shared symbolic register. In times of pandemic, such as covid-19, the public sphere is overwhelmed by an equally fast-spreading 'infodemic' (information epidemic), to borrow a term from Tedros Adhanom Ghebreyesus, director-general of the World Health Organization (who), about risk from infection and the responding collective emotional response (including repression).[38] One could see this in 2020, when there was a measurable spike in violent crimes and deaths across the United States, but this was noted only in passing in the media.[39] By reading through Kahneman and Tversky's model and emphasizing a 'positive' outcome (looking at the greater rate of infection of other social herds), one is able to stress how much less at risk *my* social herd seems to be. The lived experience of radically increased morbidity and mortality in the Other's herd would seem to negate this, however, if, as Kahneman and Tversky believe, one is acting to shape a sense of reduced risk. Risk-taking behaviour, even behaviour that seems to stress irrationality in decision-making and its perceived mitigation, would seem to favour positive outcomes for one's actions rather than negative ones. Thus one looks at the higher rates of survival rather than death within any given collective and sees that as a reason to reject any blame within the community as a form of asymmetrical risk-taking behaviour. Thus through the first year of the pandemic Trump surrogates claimed that only 1 or 2 per cent (Dr Ben Carson, Trump's Secretary of Housing and Urban Development) or at most 3.4 per cent (Senator Ron Johnson, Republican-Wisconsin) of those infected in the United States would succumb to the virus. This, on first hearing, sounded trivial. That this would have amounted to as many as 1 to 2 million deaths was a reality check on the seemingly trivial '1' per cent.

Even Jon Elster's work on *Ulysses and the Sirens*, which stresses imperfect rationality, that one is restrained from action until a fascinating 'siren' (positively or negatively) has passed, does not factor in the necessary types of projection that we observe within these communities.[40] His work on the impact of perceived availability of transplants only examines the idea of competition for transplants within a medical community context and not any given community's symbolic sense of whether such transplants are acceptable, as in the late twentieth-century debate about the use of swine organs as xenographs. Even when memory is introduced as a feature of such constructions, they fail to account for collective choice rooted in actions that are self-destructive. 'Hysterisis', according to one economic theory, is the presence of a phantom-limb effect in choice. When the actual cause of action is removed, the memory and response to the memory remain as subliminal factors.[41] Such a mechanistic view negates the persistence of affect embedded in symbolic registers, not experience, as the initial impulse for such choices, even the rejection, as we shall see later, of vaccination in the midst of the pandemic. Rational choice, even imperfect but plottable, does not provide the sort of explanatory framework to comprehend such collective responses, as there really does not seem to be the option for disinterested choice within the responses to and the projection of culpability for epidemics and pandemics. The examination of the affect upon which such choices are made provides some sense of the contingency of placing blame.

Out-groups

When early in the COVID-19 pandemic out-groups such as Muslim pilgrims or Muslims in general were accused of spreading COVID-19 – labelled 'corona jihad' – and endangering the 'innocent' in the emerging Hindu nationalist world of India, it would seem that the older model had simply recapitulated itself. Words matter: the term evoked the angry fantasy of the international conspiracy of 'love jihad', the Hindutva notion that Muslim men seduce Hindu women in order to convert them, itself a version of the anxieties that were encapsulated in laws against 'miscegenation' in nineteenth-century America or in the 1935 Nazi Nuremberg Laws banning Jews from marrying 'Aryans'. Diseases too are social phenomena. In the nineteenth century the British engagement in India spread what had been local epidemics such as cholera across the world, threatening European cities. Yet it was the non-white bodies in Asia that were blamed as the source of the disease, not local transmission and global trade.[42] In his history of Orissa, William Hunter, a British historian and civil servant working in British India, identified Hindu and Muslim pilgrimages as

> the most powerful of all the causes which conduce to the development and propagation of Cholera epidemics ...
> The devotees [pilgrims] care little for life or death, nor is it possible to protect men against themselves. But such carelessness imperils lives far more valuable than their own
> ... [Such carelessness] may any year slay thousands of the most talented and the most beautiful of our age in Vienna, London, or Washington.[43]

Hunter's proto-epidemiology established one of the early global health maps and pinpointed certain groups of people, from Hindu to Muslim pilgrims, as being responsible for the spread of devastating diseases across the world. It also resulted in Indian Muslim hajis (pilgrims) being subjected to prolonged and humiliating periods of quarantine.[44] The administration of draconian public health measures aimed at preventing spread of the epidemic disease fostered systemic tension between Hindu and Muslim communities in the Ganges delta who had previously been lumped together by the British colonial administration as 'Asian'. By the close of the nineteenth century, these would lead to global restrictions on such groups as carriers of epidemic diseases. When nineteen European nations met in Dresden on 15 April 1893 and sealed a sanitary convention, the treaty singled out for control of infectious diseases such as cholera certain categories of people, such as 'Gipsies, vagrants, [and] Emigrants, and persons passing the frontiers in numbers.'[45] In Imperial Germany, the jumping-off point of millions of East European Jews in Bremerhafen and Hamburg, the reference was clear, but the intent transcended even local interest. For the European imperial powers gathered around the table, it was also clear that it reflected official policy concerning all groups imagined as putting the homeland as well as their citizens in the colonies at risk. By attributing the disease to a foreign threat, such public health policy incited or reinforced xenophobia.

By the turn of the twenty-first century, with the radicalization of Islam in South Asia and Hindu nationalism, the racist language and attitudes of the earlier colonial power reemerged with a certain viciousness. After a meeting of the Muslim missionary society Tablighi Jamaat in Delhi led to a COVID-19 outbreak in April 2020, Hindu nationalists blamed all Muslims for the spread of the virus to innocent Hindu victims. As one Hindu nationalist interviewed at the time noted: 'These are dangerous people, these lockdown cheats. They have compromised us all.'[46] Earlier in the pandemic, Muslim pilgrims were blamed for spreading the disease around the world after the Chinese had supposedly 'contained' it.[47] That such prejudices existed in the United States because of 9/11 is well documented and yet they have not reappeared with the same vehemence with COVID-19, as the South Asian community, while also disproportionately impacted, is not under the same level of politicization as in Modi's India.[48] Yet by the spring of 2021, South Asians were included de facto in the category 'AAPI' (Asian American and Pacific Islanders) in the USA as they had been in 'BAME' (Black, Asian and minority ethnic) communities in the UK, as they were among those who were attacked as surrogates for the 'Chinese', as we shall discuss in detail in the next chapter. As the COVID-19 pandemic progressed, Saudi Arabia banned Muslim pilgrims from outside the country from going to Mecca and Medina to perform Haj – one of the basic tenets of Muslim ritual practice. This was a logical attempt to retard the spread of the virus, not an attempt to vilify other Muslims. And yet within the communities there have been radically different responses both to the outbreaks of the pandemic and to the stigmatization of these radically different Islamic communities. This had more to do with cultural history than disease aetiology.

Health and illness are always part of the symbolic register that defines a community's boundaries. Thus the very idea of the public's health is intertwined with the self-understanding and self-definition of the imagined community. Out-groups look at their image in the public sphere and try to redefine themselves as either not at risk or at less risk than other subaltern out-groups. What is vital is that each member of the group is forced to acknowledge and reinterpret the boundaries that they have generated between themselves and the greater society. No general rule can be applied if these boundaries are seen as impermeable by some and flexible by others. The rigid boundaries created by the national state in defining health as a quality of good citizenship has meant that accepting blame turns out to be virtually impossible without projecting it beyond the group. This may take the form of a structure of self-defence while casting the state as the enemy; it may take the form of seeing the state as having been infiltrated by the enemy. While it remains a cliché, the public's health even in times of peril is always political and is part of a symbolic register that has echoes in a communal sense of shared meaning. As much as lockdown or quarantine and other public health practices are necessary means of controlling epidemics and public anxiety, placing the blame is needed even when one is endangered and endangering others. As with many such public health interventions, placing blame can often inspire in some a false sense of protection through the creation of an implied boundary between one community and another, which turns out be dangerous to the public's health, for the cognitive dissonance created within such groups diverts individuals and groups from taking the appropriate precautions to guard their health. David Napier warned us in 2017 that 'there is today an especially urgent need to rethink the relationship between epidemics and xenophobia' given 'the human tendency to take bad meaning over no meaning, as Nietzsche so aptly put it, reverting to scapegoat narratives that should have no place or register in the multicultural settings that world populations increasingly inhabit'.[49] By 2020 it was clear that, augmented by the global media and social media, placing blame facilitates and enforces both the drawing of boundaries using the symbolic registers available and the identification of others to blame.[50] Not only is placing blame in times of stress triggered by social inequalities, as argued by Marxist and functionalist historians alike, but, as we learn over and over again, while public health measures, from building sanitary cordons and enforcing maritime quarantine to locking down cities and closing borders, may be necessary measures to prevent epidemics, they also build psychological obstructions and reinforce existing boundaries. They may indeed save lives, but what kind of lives? And whose? And what are the meanings that any community projects onto these lives in their symbolic world?

2

CHINA, WUHAN AND RACE

The pandemic of COVID-19 has been laid at the feet of the Chinese simply because it was first reported in the People's Republic of China (PRC) in 2019. (In the PRC COVID-19 is officially referred to as the novel coronavirus pneumonia or NCP.) Yet such a clear statement is fraught with multiple overlays of stereotypes. As of the second half of the eighteenth century, the increasingly negative perception of China in the West helped to create the image of the 'Sick man of Asia', 'the home of plague, famine, intrigue, flood, graft and corruption'.[1] The Chinese, a label often used to encompass all immigrants from East Asia, were the out-group who were seen as a source of social ills and threats to the health of White Christian society over the course of the nineteenth century. Chinese populations living on the Pacific coast of the United States as well as in Canada were regularly used as a scapegoat by local health officials for the failure of their sanitary programmes.[2] They blamed all epidemic outbreaks on the crowded living conditions among the Chinese as well as their different, hence 'primitive' and 'unclean', habits. Indeed, the politics behind the exclusion of the Chinese, as the 'Yellow Peril', from White demographics was to no little degree a factor of a pattern of eugenic thought that coupled Asians with illness.[3] In 1885 J. A. Chapleau, the Canadian Secretary of State, compared Vancouver's Chinatown to 'an ulcer lodged like a piece of wood in the tissues of the human body, which unless treated must cause disease in the places around it and ultimately to the whole body'.[4] In the United States, a series of epidemics of smallpox in the 1870s and the bubonic plague in 1900 in San Francisco were used by authorities to justify the 1882 Chinese Exclusion Acts.[5]

Today, when we turn to Nexis for citations including 'China' and that nineteenth-century trope, the 'sick man of Asia', we find well in excess of 5,300 citations after 1 March 2020. (In our study we shall be using Nexis, a database of worldwide newspapers, news transcripts, magazines and legal opinions, to measure the debates within the public sphere.) This at a time when Asian Americans were already suffering disproportionate rates of COVID-19 infection, reflecting long-term group prejudice.[6] When the *Wall Street Journal* published a piece on 4 February 2020 on the Chinese economy (not the virus) by Walter Russell Mead entitled 'China is the Real Sick Man of Asia', the blowback was strong and immediate. Readers (and the Chinese Foreign Ministry) censured the piece (or at least its title) because of its clear reference to the trope of disease and the present crisis. China revoked the press credentials of three *Wall Street Journal* reporters and condemned the title of the piece as 'racially discriminatory' and a slander on the government's 'efforts in fighting COVID-19'.[7] Harry Zhang, associate professor at Old Dominion University in Virginia, said in a letter to the *Wall Street Journal* that

> I was horrified to read the headline ... At this critical moment for millions of Chinese who are suffering from the coronavirus, this headline triggers the extremely miserable memory for the Chinese since 1840 when the First Opium War broke out. I respect the First Amendment, but in a

civilized society we should not tolerate this discriminatory
opinion while humanity is under siege.[8]

In a subsequent letter to the editor of the *International Journal of
Surgery*, a final-year medical student of Chinese ancestry, S. O.
Cheng, made the connection between past and present crystal clear, bringing anti-Asian feeling generated by COVID-19 into
the context of a canon of such moments of blaming the Other.
His central theme is that 'xenophobia has spread much like the
virus itself, affecting those not just of Chinese descent but to
those of any East Asian origin or nationality.' He frames this
experience with the statement that 'similar phenomena have
occurred in other disease pandemics; pogroms against Jewish
communities during the bubonic plague in the 14th century, stig-
matisation of the LGBTQ+ community in the HIV outbreak of the
1980s and recently, xenophobia towards African and Caribbean
communities during the 2014 Ebola outbreak.'[9] All are false; all
are pejorative; all must be rejected. Unless they happen to be
accurate.

Until January 2020 Wuhan, a mega-city with hypermodern
infrastructures from colossal road networks to high-speed railways, had served as a tangible symbol and shining example of
China's ever-growing economy as well as the country's seemingly
unstoppable rise. It had impressed visitors around the world:
the once 'Sick man of Asia' had grown to a global economic
giant.[10] Such growth was coupled by an unprecedented scale
of urbanization, driving millions of rural villagers into cities. It
was however dwarfed by a fragmented and overloaded health
system that was largely self-policing. Cities such as Wuhan con-
tinuously created greater health risks, from air pollution to flu
pandemics. Rhetorically, the Chinese authorities acknowledged

that an efficient health system was pivotal to China's overall social and economic development, the country's stability and the Communist Party's political legitimacy, as well as China's image on the world stage. As of the late 1990s, Chinese authorities had begun to introduce various health reforms, including adopting the u.s. Centers for Disease Control and Prevention (CDC) system. But the lack of financial commitment from the State Council and of resources and enthusiasm at the grassroots level meant the ambitious plans on paper were not implemented on the ground. The SARS outbreak in 2003 exposed grave deficiencies in the Chinese health system and coincided with China securing funding from the World Bank to carry out a number of ten-year public health projects to control infectious diseases. This led to the opening of new local CDCs throughout China, which replaced those old and mostly crumbling disease-control units that had been set up during the Mao era (1949–76) and lasted until 1983. Much of the money from the World Bank was used to upgrade the appropriate areas of medical science and build a high-tech Internet system for disease surveillance and reporting. Yet a systematic prevention programme remained absent.

As the political importance of SARS receded, and when the World Bank-funded public health projects came to an end, the Chinese authorities put little money and less effort into making them sustainable and developing an autonomously robust disease-control programme. The disease-control programme remained and remains largely ad hoc. It has constantly failed stress tests and was unable to cope with major disease outbreaks. In the meantime, the continuing debates in global public health over the horizontal approach versus the vertical approach to health as well as the complex legacy of the Maoist approach to health left Chinese policy-makers and public health experts struggling to come up with a model that would cope with the country's ever-growing and changing health demands.[11] Prior to 2019 the Chinese health system was already overloaded, plagued by vaccine scandals and subject to physician overcharging and frequent medical accidents. With an increasing number of dissatisfied, angry patients violently taking out their frustrations against health professionals, enrolment in medical schools had fallen sharply in recent years. The Chinese CDC that had been given the responsibility to control diseases had neither the money nor the power to implement disease control. Local health providers, who need to sustain their livelihood by making profits on their enterprises, were not obliged to comply with the CDC recommendations. At the same time, the effects of infectious disease outbreaks were often made worse by weak, vertical lines of communications between local and higher-level health bodies in China. When a frontline health worker or the local CDC reported a potential health threat, it was often dismissed, like the dead rat that Dr Rieux kicks aside in Albert Camus' *The Plague*.[12] Like most authorities, the Chinese authorities have shown repeated reluctance to accept and acknowledge a major disease outbreak because acknowledgement would threaten their political legitimacy and economic interests.

Such limitations of access run parallel to the shifts in healthcare delivery in the PRC. Since the late 1980s the PRC government has opted for a market model for financing health services. This quickly led to the problem of urban access to healthcare, where decentralized systems were inappropriate and centralized systems expensive and hence unaffordable for those displaced rural migrants in the cities. Their lack of access to urban healthcare made the majority of rural migrants more vulnerable to disease outbreaks, such as during the SARS outbreak in 2003 and more recently in Wuhan during the coronavirus outbreak. These rural migrant workers often live in squalid and crowded conditions, often with no access to clean water and washing facilities. Their workplaces became a hotbed for the spread of a number of infectious diseases well in advance of 2019.

On 8 December 2019 the first case of COVID-19 was recorded in Wuhan's hospital Internet reporting system, but it was only in late December, when the disease had begun to spread across the Chinese border, that the authorities in Hubei province (Wuhan being the capital) began slowly to acknowledge that there was community transmission happening in the city. Still, they withheld crucial information that provided clues that the virus was spreading among humans, and they failed to communicate with residents about the seriousness of the situation or to attempt to educate the public to take precautions and try to mitigate the spread of the outbreak. Unalarmed, in January thousands of families in Wuhan attended a huge celebratory banquet – a super-spreader event that helped the virus to spread rapidly and widely around the city and beyond. In the meantime, authorities silenced those health professionals such as Dr Li Wenliang who had raised the initial alarm. Local public security officers – the equivalent of the police – knocked on Dr Li's door and forced him to sign a confession to spreading 'false information'.

Indeed, in late December 2020 Zhang Zhan, one of the 'citizen journalists' who blogged from Wuhan during the lockdown, was sentenced to four years in prison for challenging the official narrative with her harrowing accounts of those isolated there. Her work had worldwide resonance as a voice from the trenches. The official court convicted her of 'picking quarrels and provoking trouble', a vague charge commonly used against critics of the government.[13] Two citizens of Wuhan who blogged about daily life in the city during the lockdown also faced threats and even in January 2021 were still being constantly monitored. Ai Xiaoming, a film-maker who called for the local authorities to be held accountable, had her account on the popular social media platform WeChat shut down. Fang Fang, the award-winning writer whose lockdown diary was translated into English and published overseas, had her publishing contracts suspended.[14] Chinese publishing houses stopped releasing her work. To admit, either within or beyond the borders of the PRC, the presence of a major disease outbreak would run the risk of social dissolution. 'Political correctness is so prioritized that when we're in a crisis, even weeping and mourning are deemed [to be] bringing shame on the country and delivering the sword to the outside world,' Fang Fang told *The Guardian*'s Michael Standaert in a recent interview.[15]

The official public health authorities as well as medical science in the PRC were never quite separate from such political considerations. While the government had seemingly provided genetic data on the virus in mid-January 2020, the reality was that it had already been leaked to a virology website by a researcher, forcing its hand. Since the WHO needed official collaboration with the PRC, public statements praising the government's actions, including by Tedros Adhanom Ghebreyesus, the director-general of the WHO, were paralleled by a raft of behind-the-scenes telephone calls coaxing officials in charge to try and get them to actually supply real-time data about infection rates and local spread.[16] By January 2021, after months of back-and-forth requests from WHO officials who wanted to visit Wuhan to begin to investigate the origin of the zoonotic spread of the virus (not the conspiratorial claims that it was created in a laboratory setting there, perhaps in concert with Bill Gates and

George Soros), the Chinese government would not grant them visas.[17] Ghebreyesus expressed his deep disappointment at the stonewalling of his investigators, two of whom were in the air when the visas were denied.[18] When queried, a Chinese foreign ministry spokeswoman avoided directly answering international press questions on the matter. While appearing polished, she would repeat the official script of obfuscations and misdirection.[19] Almost a year after the coronavirus first appeared in Wuhan it was finally admitted that there had been suppression of information about the initial outbreak. This happened only after a spectacular jump in confirmed infections to 138 per day on 13 January 2021, the highest recorded rate of daily infections following the lifting of the initial total lockdown that had begun in March 2020. On 14 January 2021 the Chinese authorities finally allowed some members of the WHO investigation team into Wuhan, some of whom had been long-term collaborators with Chinese scientists and worked on projects funded by Chinese state grants, but who then expressed pessimism that any findings would be quickly forthcoming.[20] In the meantime, official propaganda in China focused on China's transparency in sharing the information. 'China is stonewalling the WHO, it's as transparent as mud,' said Larry Gostin, the director of the WHO's collaborating centre on national and global health law. 'The [WHO] team will not have full access to samples, data, whistle-blowers or healthcare professionals. That makes it extraordinarily difficult to conduct an investigation the world can have confidence in.'[21] His was not an unfounded speculation. All thirteen members of the WHO team were sequestered in their hotel rooms undergoing mandatory quarantine. They were only allowed virtual meetings with a handful of carefully chosen local officials and scientists – some of whom had just been awarded national honours prior to the arrival of the WHO team: be loyal to the party and you will be rewarded, a mechanism the Communist Party learned from the Chinese emperors in efficiently running such a vast country. Even the eventual and limited site visits to the closed public market that was believed to have been the starting point of the outbreak were very carefully choreographed. In the meantime, however, speculation – based on work done at the State Key Laboratory of Virology, School of Health Sciences, Wuhan University, as well as at Wuhan CMLabs – intimated that the official figures not only of the initial outbreak but of the smaller outbreaks in a number of Chinese cities beginning in autumn 2020 suggested, based on massive serological studies, that SARS-CoV-2 may exist for a very long time in a population without any overt clinical cases. In other words, the official figures produced by China may well be much lower than the actual number of infections, both initially as well as in early 2021.[22]

In the current pandemic, public health scientists often make the claim that their science is not politics, but of course it always is. For public health is by definition a translational field, not from laboratory to clinic, but from laboratory or fieldwork to policy. The consequences of all policy in a pandemic/epidemic are political, beyond the field of science, as they rest on the presuppositions of the society in which such claims are made. In 2020 we saw quack claims become public policy. Thus the half-hearted quasi-approval by the U.S. Federal Drug Authority in May 2020 of hydroxychloroquine and chloroquine, advocated by Donald Trump and his minions. We also saw social interventions, such as lockdowns, that are acknowledged as appropriate become instruments of political suppression. In Hong Kong this was a means of controlling political activity in response to the new national security law imposed by the authorities in Beijing. In the border regions of the PRC disease-controlling measures were used in order to suppress minority groups such as the Uyghur Muslims in Xinjiang. Such politicization of health is nothing new and not unique to China. Gerald Geison's 1995 work on the 'private science' of Louis Pasteur in his work on rabies and anthrax as well as Susan Lederer's account of human experimentation (such as the yellow fever experiments by the Reed Commission during the Spanish-American war) are examples of how what in the end was 'good' science was shackled to the ideological goals of the experimenter.[23] As we shall discuss below, the long history of European, in particular British and French, imperial interests in the natural history and wildlife of China and Asia was part of a scientific imperialism that undergirded their colonial systems. Although the empires are gone, that imperial impulse has never totally disappeared.

Whether the infectious virus that is at the root of COVID-19 is of animal origin or not is less important, as it is in the end transmitted through our social network and cultural pathways. David Dasak, the president of EcoHealth Alliance in New York and the WHO official tasked with heading the visiting group in Wuhan in February 2021, pointed out there were much larger clusters of transmission outside of the Huanan seafood market, which was identified as the first site of the pandemic. Yet without any evidence, he pointed as potential sources to other markets where live or recently killed wildlife, such as civets (as in the SARS pandemic) or even pangolins, are said have been sold for human consumption. Since no viruses were found in any of the frozen specimens in the markets, this is clearly not 'scientific truth' but Western cultural prejudice against the eating of certain foods.[24] While Dasak praised the Chinese public health researchers and scientists in Wuhan, with whom he had earlier collaborated, for their 'openness', it was clear that the official Chinese narrative was that the virus was 'alien' and mostly likely imported from abroad through the food chain, with imported foreign frozen meat pinpointed as the potential source. The WHO team seemed to declare this a possibility at the final news conference, much to the delight of the Chinese state authorities. Even though Chinese researchers found live coronavirus on packages of frozen meat and codfish as well as signs of the virus inside packaging in different parts of China, the risk of surface transmission remained low. In all nine incidents identified by the Chinese researchers, tabulated in articles by Emanuel Goldman in *The Lancet* (1 August 2020) and Dynai Lewis in *Nature* (26 February 2021; updated 15 March 2021) it is more likely that the virus was transmitted through the huge volume of human traffic inside food markets and warehouses, not from frozen food to human. Fabian Leendertz, a German zoonotic disease specialist and a member of the team, stated that it was a 'very unlikely scenario', but that the WHO team had decided to include the frozen food theory among its hypotheses 'to respect, a bit, the findings' of their Chinese colleagues.[25] The official *Report of the WHO-China Joint Mission on Coronavirus Disease 2019 (COVID-19)* was released on 30 March 2021, with the caveats in place.

The official Report of the WHO-China Joint Mission on Coronavirus Disease 2019 (COVID-19) was released on 30 March 2021. Employing only PRC-generated data, it basically concluded that while one would probably never absolutely know how the pandemic originated, it was most likely passed from bats or pangolins to animals raised for human consumption. It also drew into question whether the Wuhan market was the pandemic's point of origin, speculating that the virus had been circulating for weeks prior to the outbreak there. The report draft also explained that the evolutionary distance between bat-based coronaviruses and sars-CoV-2 was estimated to have been several decades, 'suggesting a missing link'. It reaffirmed that the pandemic, even if it is of zoonotic origin, was rapidly transmitted from human to human. Previous cases observed outside the area of the Huanan market suggest the outbreak began elsewhere. 'No firm conclusion therefore about the role of the Huanan market in the origin of the outbreak, or how the infection was introduced into the market, can currently be drawn' wrote the investigators. One hypothesis that the origin was in imported frozen foods was deemed worthy of further study but the supposition that the virus had escaped from the Wuhan virology laboratory was dismissed out of hand. The report was heralded by Chinese state authorities as definitive and as absolving them from blame for their handling of the initial outbreak, while fourteen national governments, including the United States and United Kingdom, remained sceptical, seeing it more as a political than a scientific statement. In the end, health politics is politics. And politics have always played a crucial role in international health. As Dr Sze Szeming, one of the who's founding fathers, remembered, from the outset the who really had more to do with politics than medicine.[26]

Food Is 'Dangerous'

In Wuhan, having tried to control the information at the very beginning of the outbreak in January 2020, the authorities quickly placed the blame on the poor migrant vendors working out of the Huanan seafood market, even though only a small number of vendors were infected compared to much larger clusters of infection throughout the city. Knowing the Western world's fetishistic disgust over the Chinese and indeed Asian trade in wildlife, authorities traced the disease to the seafood market and symbolically shut down and disinfected the market, depriving those stall owners of their livelihood. This echoed the debates concerning the origin of the SARS infection, which was seen as stemming from the consumption of flesh from wild animals and led to the closing of virtually all the open-air markets in Hong Kong and the fetishistic imposition of Western standards of 'hygiene', achieved through moving the vendors into what to all intents and purposes were concrete car parks.[27]

The animal origin of SARS in 2003 was also highly contested. Was it spread by chickens and other domestic animals raised for food or by wild animals, such as civet cats, used for food?[28] It seemed to be transmitted through the food chain. Soon it was clear that 'food handlers working in Guangdong's busy markets [were] heavily represented among those who became ill with the mysterious disease.'[29] In the winter of 1997 millions of chickens had been killed and the corpses burned in Hong Kong because of the fear of a lethal avian influenza that had the potential to infect human beings.[30] As with the public discourse about obesity, food that was essential to our survival seemed to be striking back to kill us. With 813 deaths out of a total of 8,437 infectious people before SARS was declared in July 2003, SARS was touted as the next great pandemic. Even the jokes that circulated in China made this association: 'What the Party has failed to do, SARS has succeeded in doing: The party failed to control dining extravagantly. SARS did.'[31] Or the benefit a wife received from SARS: 'The husband who self-indulgently gorges on meat in restaurants, all of a sudden, turns into a rabbit and takes a fancy to the various vegetable dishes cooked at home, contending that eating vegetables may boost his immune system.'[32] And the disease itself was seen as originating in the food chain. SARS created a moral panic about the spread of infectious diseases through global travel, as the disease moved from Asia to Europe to North America. While the number of cases was limited, the powerful association of disease with the problems inherent in the food chain made pinpointing the origin of the disease in food a means of controlling the panic associated with the disease.

One can note that this specificity about the food chain and 'wild' animals is applied only to the exotic, whether it is the food consumed or the culture permitting its consumption. When Westerners arranged massive shoots to kill innumerable wild quail, pheasant and boar for their consumption in Europe or in China, this was seen as part of the civilizing process.[33] It is not actually what you eat, but the symbolic register of what you eat, that is determinant. As the anthropologist Claude Fischler argues, 'Human beings mark their membership of a culture or a group by asserting the specificity of what they eat, or more precisely – but it amounts to the same thing – by defining the otherness, the difference of others.'[34] By the time of the pandemic in 2020 the far right identified the origin and spread of the novel coronavirus as a problem inherent to Chinese civilization and its idiosyncratic eating patterns. Senator John Cornyn (Republican) of Texas supported Trump's accusation that the Chinese were solely at fault, for 'China is to blame because the culture [is] where people eat bats and snakes and dogs and things like that.' One can note that Texas is quite famous for annual 'rattlesnake roundups', where the snakes are milked for anti-venom before their meat is consumed fried as a test of masculinity.[35] What is permitted and forbidden in foodstuffs and foodways is always symbolic.

From the Hellenistic Jewish literature of the first century that has been preserved we can see that the prohibition on foreign food enabled the authors and their readers to imagine a separate Jewish identity apart from what they saw as a hostile, 'unclean' and 'unrighteous' Greco-Roman environment, equivalent to the Gentile's sexual defilement of the Jews.[36] The latter, according to Philo, was the cause of the 'female disease' among Jewish men – rendering men feminine, hence 'unfit' and shameful in a patriarchal culture that celebrated masculinity.[37] The early Church Fathers rejected biblical dietary restrictions as Noahide laws, applicable only to the Jews, by stressing that God created all food and that none should be rejected (1 Timothy 4:1–4). Early Christian authorities still imposed the prohibition of animal sacrifice as a state policy, hence also prohibiting the Greek practice of eating food after sacrifice. Again, food practices were used to demarcate Christians from the 'idolatry' of the Greeks. All such lines, from the prohibition of eating 'unclean' pork in Leviticus 11:7–8, to that of eating fava beans, which were considered impure among the Pythagoreans, had to do with abstract means of limiting risk. Mary Douglas, in her essay on the 'Abominations of Leviticus' (1966), stressed that we should not attribute a sort of medical materialism to the ancients.[38] They certainly did not know about trichinosis in pork, even though many medical thinkers, such as Sir William Osler (for whom 'Moses was the first hygienist') in the nineteenth century, assumed that they did (or at least that an omniscient God did). As for Pythagoras' fava bean fetish: as they both caused intestinal gas, and therefore, when expelled, eliminated the breath necessary for life, as well as contained the souls of the dead, they brought the boundary between life and death into the deft hands of the philosopher.[39] This is certainly more compelling than believing that the Greeks (or at least their gods) had secret knowledge of 'favism', G6PD deficiency, with its deleterious effects on red blood cells. By creating categories that limited risk, by declaring as abominations food that did not fit their strict models of the natural world, the ancients attempted to locate their fears of impurity and contamination, of health and disease. In the next centuries, food laws and practices would become one of the salient defining markers that separated Jews, Christians and Muslims.[40]

European (read: Christian) aversion to others' unfamiliar dietary practices would become exacerbated with increased contact with the non-Christian world after the fourteenth century, when the period of peace under Mongol rule allowed many Europeans to travel beyond their immediate horizon. Overwhelmed by a world so different from their own, many of them were simultaneously exhilarated and frightened by their experiences. Among these earlier European travellers were a great number of Catholic emissaries on papal missions to explore opportunities to bring Christianity to China and beyond. The East, according to some of them, was the 'tree of paradise' that at the same time was full of 'monstrous' serpents – the roots of 'the transgression of our first parents'.[41] The Portuguese Franciscan friar Odoric of Pordenone, a near contemporary of Marco Polo of Venice, was sent to the East on papal business and travelled extensively across Mongol-ruled China for three years beginning in 1320. In the southern port city of Canton, he marvelled at the abundance and wide variety of high-quality foods available but also noted, 'here too, there be serpents bigger than anywhere else in the world, many of which are taken and eaten with relish. These serpents [have quite a fragrant odour and] form a dish so fashionable that if a man were to give a dinner and not have one of these serpents on his table, he would be thought to have done nothing.'[42] Odoric's account circulated widely in manuscript: at least a hundred manuscript copies survived and were plagiarized in the widely read fourteenth-century English romance *The Voyage and Travels of Sir John Mandeville, Knight*. Odoric's amazement at the novel culinary delights of inhabitants of southern China horrified some English and European readers, however. The adjective 'monstrous' would be added to the noun 'serpents' in a number of translations. (However, the French sinologist Jacques Gernet, who has used these and other Chinese sources, points out that these were not serpents but brushwood eels, which are still a culinary delight consumed in China today.[43] Eels and elvers were and remain widely consumed throughout Western Europe too, of course.[44]) As of the fifteenth century, with the advent of European and British expansions to new and unknown territories, the perception that there were growing rates of illness among European settlers caused by the hot (rendered as 'unhealthy') climates in the south was viewed as a barrier to European expansion as well as a drain on manpower.[45] At the same time, a growing number of accounts in both popular and medical literature began to paint an image of such newly acquired lands, seen as culturally alien and environmentally distinct, as 'tropics' filled with beasts and naked men who consumed human flesh and who lived among snakes and lizards while transmitting horrifying diseases. These accounts contributed to the shifting image of the tropics from an earthly paradise to a terrestrial hell.[46] Such dark images of the tropics as the place where diseases originated would harden in the nineteenth century, when accelerated engagement in colonies across several continents brought epidemic diseases such as cholera (labelled 'Asian cholera') to European cities, thereby threatening White populations.

The new discipline of 'tropical diseases', developed as part of the 'white man's burden' to make colonial subjects into worthwhile labourers and preserve the health of colonial settlers, emerged to fuel imperial ambition and expansion. The tropics, 'divided equally between jungle, tigers, cobras, cholera and sepoys', had to be tamed and transformed by White Europeans with their modern bio-medicine and hygiene.[47] When the advances of European bio-medicine failed to conquer diseases that continue to ravage the tropics to this day, such as malaria and schistosomiasis, and with the rise of germ theory at the close of the nineteenth century, they placed blame on the Asians for their 'dirty' and 'primitive', hence 'unhygienic', habits and their dietary practice of eating raw, wild foods such as field snails, even though the affluent and 'civilized' Europeans continued to swallow oysters raw as a culinary delight and aphrodisiac, and wild ones were considered 'healthier'.[48] Asians were also accused of being the villains in the slaughter and trade in wild animals, even though they were not the only ones who participated in the ever-growing maritime fur trade. Indeed, the debate about the massive slaughter of seals in the Arctic for fashionable clothing during the 1890s led to a confrontation between Britain, the United States, France and Russia about the potential extermination of pelagic seals, resulting in a compact in 1893, one of the few attempts until the late twentieth century to stop the eradication of a species.[49] Animals matter; diseases did not and do not respect the assumed boundaries between the objects of trade and consumption and those doing the trading and consuming.

The ideology that links food and illness is the antithesis of that which demands that food and diet are the cure for disease. In late nineteenth-century America these two forces paralleled one another, much as they did in Chinese Medicine or indeed in classical Greco-Roman medicine. The muckrakers, the journalists who sought to expose corruption and bring about reform in the 'Gilded Age', stressed food as the aetiology of a range of diseases, as Upton Sinclair, one of the most effective muckrakers, did in his condemnation of the horrors of the Chicago slaughterhouses *The Jungle* (first published as a magazine serial in 1905). He described not only the unsanitary scenes in the abattoirs but the skin diseases that resulted from the exposure to the picking room and men with tuberculosis spitting and coughing on the processing line. He detailed how rotten and infected meat was reprocessed and sold, passing infections on to the public. This image, multiplied a thousandfold in the popular literature of the day, contributed in 1906 to the passage of the Pure Food and Drug Act. But this act excepted 'health supplements' from any oversight. These were continued to be marketed as health interventions, even if they were ineffective or produced unknown and often negative side effects. On the other hand, Dr John Harvey Kellogg's sanitarium in Battle Creek, Michigan, developed a wide range of 'health foods', following the vegetarian tradition of the Seventh-Day Adventists, so that by 1900, his brother William's 'Corn Flakes' (1894) and the creations of his followers such as C. W. Post (with the coffee substitute 'Postum' in 1895) had become standard household brands, encouraging 'healthy' eating. Here one can note that brother William broke with John over his desire to add sugar to make the product more marketable (but, of course, less 'healthy'). For social hygienists food and health/illness are seen to be intimately linked. That diseases from animals could infect humans was obvious to the readers of *The Jungle*, but it was just as evident to them that yellow fever was spread by mosquitos (claimed by Carlos Finlay in 1881 but only publicly confirmed by the Walter Reed Commission in 1900). Such health risks really were ubiquitous.

Stereotypes place the blame for pandemics on exotic peoples in the tropics consuming disgusting foods; but disease, of course, can be spread to people from animals whether they are domesticated or wild. Zoonotic diseases are transmitted from animals to humans, and stem from bacterial, viral, parasitic or fungal infection of an animal host that spreads to humans through bites, scratches or ingestion. They are known throughout the world and have impacted human health throughout history.[50] Similarly, some so-called 'tropical' diseases, such as malaria, were indigenous in Europe well into the twentieth century (and reappeared with a vengeance after the collapse of the USSR). While malaria has ceased, at least for the time being, to be a public health problem in the West, a number of newly emerged zoonotic diseases are presenting increasing threats to the West owing to growing contact and trade between the West and the rest of the world. In the meantime, with the growing anxiety over the loss of wildlife, a mixed legacy of earlier European expansion and post-Second World War development projects as well as population growth, China and other developing Asian countries have been targeted by Western wildlife conservation organizations, even though the natural paradise imagined by Europeans never existed in China. It is no accident that the logo of the very Western World Wide Fund for Nature (WWF) is the giant panda. Yet it is also clear that the problem of loss of wildlife in the United States and Europe is as bad if not worse than in parts of Asia.

In the meantime, in China, rapid modernization accompanied by unrestricted deforestation and unprecedented scales of urbanization have threatened the capacity and resilience of the country's ecosystems. The ever-increasing human efforts to exploit land, from agricultural expansion and intensification – including an animal husbandry industry focused on the production of high-protein foods for human consumption given the rise in living standards – to the construction of roads, railways, mining and other large-scale modernization projects such as the Three Gorges Dam (just a little over 300 km (185 mi.) west of Wuhan), contributed to a loss of habitats that drove much wildlife into populated areas. This led to closer contact between livestock and wildlife. It has also increased human exposure to new pathogens that threaten the public's health. South of Yangtze, including the regions around Wuhan, as well as China's southwest, has become a 'golden triangle', the ideal environment for the emergence and transmission of a number of infectious diseases, from SARS to the highly pathogenic avian influenza (HPAI) and COVID-19, all of which are zoonotic in origin. Fully aware of the problem, the Chinese government has done little to mitigate the risks, and has made little effort to educate the public about such present dangers. Yet in December 2019, to cover up for the country's mismanaged health system, they did not hesitate to reenact the nineteenth-century Western racist rhetoric that was used by American authorities to justify the Chinese Exclusion Acts of 1882, and placed the blame on those 'greedy' Chinese traders' 'dirty habit' of trade in wildlife as well as overcrowded market stalls and their vendors' unhygienic practices.[51]

The Novel Coronavirus

Having identified the supposed danger, what remains is to dispel it through a collective exorcism that involves political propaganda or moral acts mixed with forms of public health intervention.[52] Two weeks had passed in 2020 and the Chinese New Year was approaching, when millions would be on the move, potentially spreading the virus across the entire country and even the globe. Then, the central authority in Beijing grasped that the failure to control COVID-19 would cost them their political legitimacy and damage China's global image. The state authorities quickly launched a political campaign to combat the disease. China's highest political body, the Central Political and Legal Affairs Commission, not the CDC, gave the order to lock down Wuhan, a city of over 11 million. Mass lockdowns provided a feared yet politically compelling administrative option. When the lockdown in Wuhan proved impotent in stopping the virus spreading to other Chinese provinces and beyond China's borders, the authorities proceeded to close all borders and increased the level of surveillance and police power within China, targeting those disputed and troublesome border regions such as Xinjiang in the northwest, Yunnan in the southwest and Fenghe in the northeast, where systemic repression of minorities had already begun in earnest well in advance of the outbreak in Wuhan. The geographic location of the blame-game would gradually move from Wuhan to these border regions inhabited by ethnic minorities as well as to beyond the borders of the PRC.

On 7 February 2020, with the entire population of China locked indoors, Dr Li Wenliang, one of the original whistleblowers, tragically died after being infected by the virus. This event initially raised hope among many for political changes in China, a hope that was quickly crushed by an intense propaganda campaign by the official media, coupled with even tighter control of information. Anyone who put up posts about COVID-19 that contradicted the official narrative on social media platforms such as WeChat ran the risk of having their account being closed or even being arrested by the Public Security.[53] On 26 February *The Lancet* received a letter from Chinese medical officials asking the journal to retract their earlier appeal for international medical assistance to fight the COVID-19 outbreak in Wuhan. The initial appeal by physicians on the front line, made on 24 January, had suggested how devastating the situation was in Wuhan's health sectors: 'The conditions and environment here in Wuhan are more difficult and extreme than we could ever have imagined,' the authors wrote, and 'in addition to the physical exhaustion, we are also suffering psychologically. While we are professional nurses, we are also human. Like everyone else, we feel help-lessness, anxiety, and fear.'[54] The retraction came at a moment when the authorities were turning the fight against COVID-19 into a mass politicized public health campaign, and the official narrative began to paint a picture of national triumph.

The escalating pandemic around the world and many Western countries' failures to control their local transmission was contrasted with China's purported success. A catalyst for this nationalist propaganda campaign was the increasingly xeno-phobic anti-Chinese discourse in some Western countries and the anti-China campaign waged by the Republican administra-tion in the United States, which was aimed at diverting voters' attention away from the Trump administration's local misman-agement of the now exploding community transmission.[55] It allowed the official propaganda in China to turn COVID-19 into a menace from abroad. Food is central to the symbolic register long used in xenophobic discourse against the Chinese. It was utilized as a defence against the aetiology of the coronavirus in unhygienic Chinese food by the PRC authorities who argued that the virus actually had been imported into China via frozen for-eign foods. Hence COVID-19 became the new 'opium plague' that the West, in particular the United States, was using to hobble China's global rise. (In China the Opium Wars of 1839–42 and

1856–60 continue to serve as the supreme reminder of how the British imperialists enforced a shameful trade in opium, which reduced China to a state of opium slavery as Britain gradually extended its control over various ports in China. In the official historiography the opium plague had turned China into a nation of hopeless addicts, smoking themselves to death while their civilization descended into chaos.[56]) By evoking the memory of this 'national humiliation' that China had suffered under the Western imperialists, the Communist Party of China (CCP) waged a psychological war. It succeeded in rallying support from a large section of the population in China as well as overseas Chinese. The war on COVID-19 has become the twenty-first century's new opium war: never forget the humiliating past China suffered under the Western powers; we must unite together to fight external threats. As a phoenix rises from the ashes, the 'Sick man of Asia' has emerged 'triumphantly' as the official media focused on how under the CCP leadership and President Xi, China had become the global leader in the battle against the deadly virus. Vaccine nationalism was on the rise. On 8 October 2020 the PRC became the first major world economy to pledge massive support for the globalization of a COVID-19 vaccine through COVAX when it was developed. China again publicized its medical expertise in such a way as to be seen as coming to the aid of underdeveloped economies, as it did with the exportation of the 'Barefoot doctors' scheme in the 1970s.[57]

COVID-19 Spreads

In the United States, American public health authorities labelled COVID-19 the 'Wuhan virus' in January 2020 as it traced the origin of the disease, not surprisingly, to the overcrowded central

Chinese city and its dark, damp and filthy seafood market as well as the Chinese's 'despicable' habit of trading in and consuming wild animals. The same nineteenth-century rhetoric of the then cutting-edge racial sciences was brought back to life in the twenty-first century. At the very same moment, Donald Trump trumpeted the success of 'Phase One' trade talks with the PRC and soon thereafter congratulated the Chinese leadership for their handling of the spreading infection.[58] As the trade deals faded into failure and thus obscurity, and COVID-19 decimated the American economy months later, Trump loudly blamed the spread of the 'Wuhan virus', the 'China virus' or 'Kung flu' in the United States on the ineptitude or malevolence of the Chinese government. Globally, as a variety of interests intersected to replicate the horror of the pandemic in different contexts, the blame fell on the 'Chinese' (labelled 'Patient Zero', as in the alleged 'drug pandemic' that plagued the globe in the early twentieth century), and more broadly, anyone with 'yellow' skin colour who looked 'Oriental', seeming randomly to include people of East Asian and Southeast Asian heritage. In Paris at the end of February 2020 the Yuki Japanese Restaurant located in the rue de La Michodière was spray-painted with the words 'coronavirus' and 'virus' in large letters.[59] Elsewhere:

> Chinese people in Italy had likewise been discriminated against and stigmatized. Italians deserted Chinese owners' stores and restaurants. To keep their businesses open, some Chinese shop owners even let their Italian employees run them. A friend of mine saw a sign in a shop window that read: 'Every nation is able to take care of its own problems . . . It does not matter how hard it is. But in light of the fear of the corona virus, we have put

management of our store entirely in the hands of our Italian team members.'[60]

Data released under the American Freedom of Information Act also shows that there were 261 hate crimes against Asians in April 2020, rising to 323 in May, 395 in June and 381 in July 2020. Attacks on Asian Americans had spiked since the beginning of the pandemic, beginning in March 2020 and continuing to rise through January 2021, reaching over 3,000, including multiple fatal attacks on 'Asians' on both the west and the east coast as well as in the deep South.[61] That some of these Asians were Thai, Korean or Filipino as well as Chinese Americans points to the xenophobic nature of the attacks, which were aimed as an imaginary category easily filled by a wide range of individuals.[62] Russell Jeung, a professor of Asian American studies at San Francisco State University, noted that 'we're getting reports now from our reporting center. And 10, 15% of the reports are about physical assault of people getting either physically attacked or being spat upon or coughed at.' According to Metropolitan Police data, 21 attacks against 'Orientals' across Britain were recorded in January 2020 alone. This number rose steeply as the pandemic spread. While it fell during the lockdown, after the easing of restrictions in May, violence against people of East and Southeast Asian heritage started to rise steadily, reaching fifty incidents in June and sixty in July. 'It feels like the atmosphere after 9/11 towards Muslims, when any Muslim on the street was seen as a potential terrorist. Now any Chinese is . . . a potential existential threat to civilization,' says Lu Gram, a researcher at University College London who spearheaded a group called 'End the Virus of Racism'.[63] Recognizing that this category is heterogenous, from Korean Americans to Native Hawaiian Pacific Islanders in the United States and from South Asians to Chinese nationals in the UK, it is also clear that many in this overarching group suffered a disproportionate rate of morbidity and mortality from the pandemic.

In April 2020, as Wuhan as well as most of China gradually came out of the lockdown, large sections of the Chinese population began to face the grim reality of an economic recession and increased levels of social inequality. The lockdown had deprived millions of their livelihood as well as their psychological well-being. Competing for resources, lacking support, fearing the continuing pandemic and driven by the official discourse that focused on COVID-19 as a menace imported from outside, there was a greater need to place the blame for the pandemic. Racism mainly targeting African populations as well as some Muslim groups living in China – many of the former had come to China under the illusion of 'friendship' offered by the Chinese government to those 'Third World' countries after the Cold War – had been on the rise. In China, placing blame had indeed become a double-edged sword.

Who Do You Blame When You Are Blamed?

From the late nineteenth century the language of race has been an integral part of nationalistic discourse in China.[64] Armed with then-fashionable Social Darwinism, the founders of the Chinese revolution such as Sun Yat-sen argued that racial nationalism was the only vehicle capable of unifying the Chinese people and saving China from 'national humiliation'. In their nationalistic project of making China strong again, it was believed that the Chinese population – conceived as the Han race – must be taught how to be modern citizens so that they would be able to participate in this 'Dream of a Strong China'. (This would be revived in the twenty-first century by the current leadership under President Xi, except that this Chinese Dream would extend to include Africa.[65]) The modern Chinese citizen, accordingly, would have a nationalistic consciousness and at the same time live a clean and orderly life fit for a modern nation. (This was no different among the Jewish Enlighteners in Eastern Europe, for whom the health of 'ghetto Jews' was the key to their becoming full citizens, and for Zionists such as Theodor Herzl and Max Nordau at the turn of the twentieth century, who argued for a 'New Muscle Jew'.[66]) In other words, a strong, modern Chinese nation would consist of a healthy, politically enlightened and productive population. Eugenics was cherry-picked by the new Nationalist government, the first modern republic in Asia, as a solution to China's multitudinous social problems. It was believed that practising racial improvement would enable the Han/Chinese race to survive and strive.[67] Even after the West had gradually abandoned eugenics in the wake of the racial genocide committed in Nazi-ruled Europe, the then newly founded PRC continued to implement selective breeding by giving it the post-war public health label of 'family planning' or 'quality birth control'. The PRC's public health and population experts, many of whom had been trained in the United States or the Soviet Union, saw selective breeding as a means of controlling population growth which allowed them to gloss over the complex historical ethnic tensions that had begun under the Qing (Manchu) empire during the eighteenth century.

After the Manchu took over China in the 1640s, it first imposed categories of Qi (the eight banners which defined the Manchu military) and Min (all non-Manchu civilians) to separate the original Manchu units from the rest of the population.

As the Qing empire grew ever larger, by the eighteenth century including what is now called Xinjiang and Tibet in Central Asia as well as Taiwan in Southeast Asia, the Qing court moved to impose formal demarcations among the different peoples living in various parts of this colossal empire, largely for legal and tax purposes. In the eyes of the Qing emperors and the court, the Han, the name first used by some Central Asian nomadic groups for anyone who lived along their southern frontier, was only one ethnic category among many others. It was only in the late nineteenth century that Chinese nationalist thinkers, many of whom were southerners who remained loyal to the previous Ming dynasty and rejected the Qing order, called for an ideal China out of an organic relationship between their imagined state China and the Chinese people. The latter, according to them, were the Han. And for them, the Han was no longer an ethnic category but a race.[68]

After the Chinese Communist Party (CCP) became the new ruler of this vast empire originally created by the Manchus, it adopted the Soviet and Eastern European ethnic model of nationhood, with an emphasis on heredity or community of birth and (native) culture. China was reconfigured into a multi-ethnic state, with the Han as the majority ethnic group and the rest of the population divided into 56 minority groups who would become the permanent underclass or subalterns, often depicted in the official discourse as backward-thinking, ignorant, primitive, unhealthy, superstitious and needing to be enlightened through the socialist cultural revolution. Race, culture and class were conflated. Public health interventions centred on allopathic medicine that included family planning and were used as tools to bring the socialist cultural revolution into these communities, thus enforcing political hegemony and consolidating the CCP's control in these regions.[69]

As part of the public health education and family planning programme, Chinese citizens have been taught that it is for the greater good of the whole society and their patriotic duty to practise 'healthful' marriage and 'superior' birth. When this is translated into lay language, it becomes one's duty to choose a 'genetically' intelligent and healthy partner. In popular discourse, Chinese peasants, together with Chinese citizens of ethnic minorities who have darker skins as well as Blacks – the latter had traditionally been viewed in China as semi-human hovering on the edge of bestiality – were often depicted as racially inferior. Their inferiority was often 'evidenced' by their 'superstitious', translated as unscientific, practices and 'unclean' habits, but was also marked by their darker skin. In 1995 a eugenic law was officially adopted in the PRC. Forced sterilization as well as discrimination against disabled people and anyone with so-called hereditary diseases was legalized to ensure the 'physical well-being of the nation' and the 'quality of future generations'. The definition of 'disability', however, is less clear. It could apply equally to anyone who was considered too short or to have 'low intelligence'. Dubious scientific studies have been carried out suggesting that 'barbaric' marriage and reproductive habits as well as the unhealthy lifestyle of Chinese peasants, minority ethnic groups and Blacks from Africa, determined their 'genetic limitation'.[70]

While in the PRC, from the Mao era to the current leadership, the political implications of its commitment to African nations have been ever more evident, coupled with China's increasing dependence on African raw materials and the commercial importance of a potential African market, Black people have continued to be placed at the bottom of the racial/genetic hierarchy in the official and popular discourse. In southern port cities such as Guangzhou, which historically had large Muslim and Black communities and which boasts one of China's oldest mosques, there has been a growing number of African as well as Muslim (mostly from Southeast Asia) immigrants. As their forerunners did, they came to Guangzhou because it offered attractive commercial and employment opportunities. For the very same reason, Guangzhou also drew a huge number of internal migrants from all over China. The latter's lack of access to urban welfare, from housing to healthcare, as well as the discrimination many of them suffered from the existing urban population, who blamed these new migrants for competing for resources as well as making 'their' city dirty, thus unhealthy, led to some taking out their grievances against African and Muslim migrants from abroad.[71] This was made worse by authorities who blamed many of the existing societal problems on Africans and on Southeast Asian Muslims living in China: they brought the drug problem to China; they brought diseases from AIDS to swine flu – known in China as African swine flu – to China; they brought prostitution and the resultant explosion of STIs to China. When the Western world mocked China for its counterfeit goods, the Chinese authorities blamed this on Africans: it was not 'we' but 'they' who flooded the global market with fake goods and spoiled our image. In the wake of 9/11, when the West began to wage a 'war against terror', China joined the rally to label all Muslim groups, from the Uyghur in China's northwest to immigrants from different parts of Southeast Asia, as terrorists, even though these groups shared no common language (except for their children being compulsorily schooled in Mandarin – the official language of the PRC) or culture, and indeed practised very different strands of Islam. In a 2017 recommendation to the Chinese government on cracking down on Black African immigrants and traders in Guanzhou, Pan Qinglin, a member of the Chinese Political Consultative Conference – the political advisory body of the PRC – argued that Black Africans brought many security and health risks:

> [the Blacks] travel in droves; they are out at night out on the streets, nightclubs, and remote areas. They engage in drug trafficking, harassment of women, and fighting, which seriously disturbs law and order in Guangzhou ... Africans have a high rate of AIDS and the Ebola virus that can be transmitted via body fluids ... If their population [keeps growing], China will change from a nation-state to an immigration country, from a yellow country to a black-and-yellow country.[72]

On different Chinese social media platforms, people overwhelmingly supported Pan's recommendation. One commenter called on Chinese people to prevent letting 'Chinese blood become polluted'.

As of late March 2020 the official media campaign to propagate China's victory over COVID-19 had grown ever louder and was coupled by the Ministry of Foreign Affairs and National Immigration Administration's announcement to temporarily suspend the entry of foreign nationals holding valid Chinese visas or residential permits. Chinese authorities in Guangzhou launched a campaign to forcibly test Africans for COVID-19 and ordered them to quarantine in designated hotels. Chinese landlords also began to evict African residents, forcing many to sleep on the street. In the meantime, as hotels, shops, restaurants and even taxis turned away African customers, so too did the city's hospitals.[73] Elsewhere in China, there have been reports of Africans and immigrants from Southeast Asia, many of them students funded by the Chinese government to study in China, being harassed by the police and the local Chinese population. In the meantime, Pan Qinglin's 2017 recommendation has been re-circulating on Chinese social media platforms such as WeChat, fuelling popular nationalism. 'Look at them. They don't wash themselves, and they smell. They are so dirty and as black as charcoal.' 'They are crowding together again, while WE are keeping social distance. WE have worked so hard to control the virus, but they will spread it and contaminate OUR city again,' people complained. 'Tell them to go away,' some cried in their WeChat comments.

> They form, on their arrival, a community within a community, separate and apart, a foreign substance within but not of our body politic, with no love for our laws or institutions; a people that cannot assimilate and become an integral part of our race and nation. With their habits of overcrowding, and an utter disregard for all sanitary laws, they are a continual menace to health.

These last views, however, are not from WeChat but from the 1902 *Report of the Canadian Royal Commission on Chinese and Japanese Immigration*.[74] Once more, the early rhetoric used by the North American authorities to justify their racial policies against the Chinese immigrants has been re-appropriated by the in-group, the Chinese in this context, to project their own anxieties and misfortunes on to the visible but imagined out-group, Africans, and Muslims with darker skin. Like nationalism, racism has a life of its own, and can be constantly recreated and reappropriated, adapted for diverse contemporary political uses.

3

COVID-19 IN ULTRA-ORTHODOX JEWISH COMMUNITIES

O ne of the tropes that arose with COVID-19, as we noted in Chapter One, is that specific out-groups have been unfairly targeted as bearing the responsibility for the pandemic. The analogy drawn in the mass media over and over again for such a flawed and destructive attribution has been most often to the Black Death, a bubonic plague pandemic that raged in Europe from 1348 to 1351, which was blamed on the Jews. The Jews, by causing the plague, 'intended to kill and destroy the whole of Christendom and have lordship over the world', claimed a commentator in 1348 as Jews were 'dragged from their houses and thrown into bonfires'.[1] They poisoned 'rivers and fountains / That were clear and clean / They poisoned in many places,' according to the court poet Guillaume de Machaut.[2] These charges led to massive persecutions and deaths among a group already suffering and dying of the plague as much as their non-Jewish neighbours, no matter the contemporary claims for Jewish 'immunity' from infection as the basis for the antagonism against Jewish communities.[3] Indeed a simple Nexis search for the year from 1 March 2020 to 1 March 2021 turns up well over 1,600 citations for 'Jews' and 'Black Death', showing a radical increase over the course of 2020, with virtually all the media essays evoking such false attributions as *the* analogy to placing blame wrongly. Attacks on Jews as the carriers of, the cause of, the focus of COVID-19 were dismissed as a version of the hoary myth about the Black Death.[4]

Thus Mark Hay in *The Daily Beast* (online, 8 September 2020) notes the appearance of a right-wing meme advocating infecting Jews with the virus. It read: 'COVID-19. If you have the bug, give a hug. Spread the flu to every Jew. Holocough.' He comments that: 'A report by the Community Security Trust, a British group that works to stop the spread of anti-Semitism, cast the meme as the apex of far-right chatter "about getting infected, either deliberately or accidentally, and then going to synagogues and other Jewish buildings to try to infect as many Jewish people as possible".' In this context he noted that

> anti-Semitic pandemic conspiracy theories and hate had already been burbling up online for months. Conspiracy theories typically form and spread in times of confusion and upheaval, as people search for clear and easy answers, and for individuals to blame. They often pile on to estab- lished scapegoats – like Jewish populations, who have been wrongly blamed for pandemics since at least the 14th century Black Death, and falsely accused of manipulating literally every major global event to benefit themselves and hurt others.[5]

The myth framed most discussions of the false attribution of the virus to any group. From India on 10 August 2020, Jayita Mukhopadhyay wrote in *The Statesman*: 'In medieval Europe, the Jews were blamed for incurring God's wrath thought to be causing the black death and in a similar way, certain communities have been blamed for the corona outbreak both in India and in other countries, thereby spreading other deadly viruses of super- stition, prejudice, irrational hatred and concomitant violence.'[6] And we have seen in the prior chapter how the medical student

S. O. Cheng easily made this connection in his account of anti-Asian prejudice during the pandemic. (In many Southeast Asian countries, the 'Jew' and the 'Chinese' are interchangeable, pejorative categories.[7]) Don't blame the Jews for spreading infection, the trope now goes: they were the innocent victims then (and even more so now) and should not be targeted.

The Jews were not, of course, the only traditional out-group blamed for spreading the pandemic, but they have been the one that has been most articulate in claiming that stereotyping of their communities was grounded only in historical animus; indeed, rooted in antisemitic tropes of the Middle Ages.[8] While the accusation that Jews poisoned wells and caused the Black Death during the fourteenth century reappears often in the general discussion of COVID-19, only to be dismissed, it is also clear that today's ultra-Orthodox Jews (Haredim) in New York City, Israel and parts of the United Kingdom have been accused of spreading the COVID-19 virus.[9] And that charge does seem to have substance. In Rockland County, an hour's drive from New York City, which has the highest per capita rate of Jews of any American county (more than 34 per cent of the county's residents identify as Jewish), a funeral of a rabbi murdered during a home invasion at the beginning of April 2020 was labelled as a super-spreader event and Jews were seen as the source of local infections well beyond their community.[10] But, as we shall see, the charges were greater than the specific event, as Yossi Gestetner, co-founder of the Orthodox Jewish Public Affairs Council, observed: 'People in the rest of the country are blaming New York for the nationwide problem, so then people in New York are trying to blame someone else . . . But those who don't understand that . . . went out of their way to stalk, harass and discriminate against members of the community.'[11]

The Jewish communities are thus categorized as inherently different from all others, with higher rates of infection and less concern for the public's health. The underlying assumption is that the motivation is what Theodor Adorno and his colleagues Else Frenkel-Brunswik, Daniel Levinson and E. Nevitt Sanford, writing in 1950 in their now classic study *The Authoritarian Personality*, identified as 'stereotyped negative opinions describing the Jews as threatening, immoral, and categorically different from non-Jews, and of hostile attitudes urging various forms of restriction, exclusion, and suppression as a means of solving "the Jewish problem"'.[12] Not we, but our accusers, are at fault, as we are the universal victim.

The Complexity of Accuracy in Ultra-Orthodox Jewish Communities

Leading up to the economic pause caused by the pandemic, much of the secular population in Israel saw the ultra-Orthodox as the cause of the virus spreading. In April 2020 Israeli police sealed off key intersections and the army was called in to support residents of Bnei Brak when as many as 38 per cent of the 200,000 residents were infected with coronavirus, significantly higher than the national average.[13] The town was declared a 'restricted zone'. As ultra-Orthodox Jews make up a sizeable majority of the town's population, their communities were overwhelmingly impacted by the virus. Together with the Israeli Arab population in urban areas, Haredim were seen as the major source for the spread of COVID-19.[14] However, only the Haredim were viewed as 'super-spreaders' by the media at home and abroad.

Likewise, in New York City in April, restraints on the ultra-Orthodox community, whose death rates had spiked, were imposed, only to be flouted by many of the ultra-Orthodox, who attended a funeral for Rabbi Chaim Mertz in mass numbers. 'There is not a single Hasidic family that has been untouched,' said a member of the community; 'it is a plague on a biblical scale.'[15] With over seven hundred deaths among them by the autumn of 2020, touching a wide range of families, coronavirus had certainly plagued the community.[16] The mayor of New York City, Bill de Blasio, a longtime ally of the city's ultra-Orthodox, confronted local leaders. Warning that 'my message to the Jewish community, and all communities, is this simple: the time for warnings has passed,' he stated that any violation of the social distancing guidelines would lead to a summons or an arrest. He was then excoriated by Jonathan Greenblatt, the head of the Anti-Defamation League, who wrote on Twitter that 'the few who don't social distance should be called out – but generalizing against the whole population is outrageous especially when so many are scapegoating Jews. This erodes the very unity our city needs now more than ever.'[17] All Jews or just some Jews; all people or just some people. Language matters, as we shall see.

By 22 September 2020 the pandemic, which had flattened radically in New York City, was spiking again in the ultra-Orthodox Hasidic neighbourhoods of Williamsburg, Midwood, Borough Park and Bensonhurst in Brooklyn – as well as in Kew Gardens and Edgemere-Far Rockaway in Queens. The positive rates were twice what they were elsewhere in the city. The city health department warned: 'This situation will require further action if noncompliance with safety precautions is observed.'[18] Noncompliance with basic practices demanded during the pandemic, such as masking and social distancing, especially during the opening of religious schools and the High (Jewish) Holiday celebrations, were seen as the cause of the spike. The *New York*

Times, however, also referred to earlier breaches of public health concerns in this context: 'the Health Department has faced skepticism and sometimes defiance from the Hasidic community as public health officials responded to a measles outbreak and to sporadic herpes cases linked to a circumcision ritual.'[19] The reaction to the former was initially hostile.[20] The accusation that porcine gelatine was used in the preparation of the MMR vaccines exacerbated the general anti-vaccination sentiment present in the greater society and led to initial hesitation and in some cases rejection of the evident need to protect their own children from greater harm.[21] Vaccine hesitancy, growing among Jewish as well as non-Jewish middle-class communities across the United States, thus had a specific resonance in these communities. The symbolic references were different; the community responses identical. We shall return in detail to the case of herpes later on in this chapter.

Nazis

In September 2020 a second potential lockdown was thought to be possible, specifically in the Orthodox neighbourhoods of Brooklyn. With the High Holidays leading to larger gatherings, both in synagogues and in private homes, anxiety about a spike in New York City became the topic of the day. Public health officials began to leaflet these neighbourhoods with pamphlets in Yiddish and English warning about the risks for extensive community transmission. On 25 September 2020 a community meeting was chaired by NYC Health Commissioner Dave A. Chokshi, who described the recent uptick in transmission across parts of Brooklyn and Queens as 'the most precarious moment since we came out of lockdown'. The crowd consisted, among others, of a large group of ultra-Orthodox Jews opposed to both vaccination and mask-wearing, labelling the pandemic a hoax. It was led by the Orthodox radio shock-jock and candidate for City Council Heshy Tischler, wearing a 'Trump for President' button, who screamed at those speaking: 'Your violent Nazi storm troopers are coming in here to violate us. That's all you're here for!'[22] Here the pandemic scepticism represented by President (and candidate) Donald J. Trump became part of the idea constituting a community 'resistance' to state and local authority. The meeting degenerated into a verbal free-for-all, but central was the idea that the hoax was directed against the Jews and a sign of 'anti-Semitic bias on the part of public health officials confronting a real, measurable spike in infections in this community. By September 2020 a quarter of all new infections were to be found there, infections that had already claimed the lives of over 700 individuals.'[23]

In early October 2020 Tischler reappeared in a violent mass demonstration against the re-imposition by Andrew Cuomo, the governor of New York, of a partial lockdown for houses of worship because of rapid spikes in infection in, among other places, Borough Park, Brooklyn. Some participants attacked the governor for using '"irresponsible and pejorative" rhetoric'.[24] Cuomo had used a ten-year-old stock photograph of a Hasidic funeral during the news conference announcing the lockdown to illustrate the dangers existing within this community and to show why others beyond Brooklyn were at risk. During this demonstration a proponent of masking and social distancing from within the community attempted to remonstrate with the crowd. He was pelted with rocks until he became unconscious and needed to be hospitalized. What is central is that he was shouted down by the crowd as a 'Moyser', a traitor, betraying the very nature of what they considered to be central to their community identity, and thus deserving of being stoned. The excoriation took a further aggressive turn when a Yiddish-speaking photographer for a local Jewish newspaper covering the scene was shouted down: 'These were members of my own community with hatred in their eyes, flipping the finger toward me, calling me a Nazi, saying I deserve to die.'[25] While it was Cuomo who locked down the ultra-Orthodox community, de Blasio's competing attempt simultaneously to rein in the explosion of cases meant the venom was aimed at the mayor as well, who was seen as an agent of a disabled and racially inferior underclass. Tischler attacked Chirlane McCray, the wife of Bill de Blasio, as 'retard woman, coon, whatever you are'.[26] While the health department officials were the new Nazis persecuting the Jews, according to Tischler, the ultra-Orthodox were themselves certainly better than other out-groups impacted by the pandemic, such as Blacks!

On Wednesday, 6 January 2021, a mass insurrection against the federal government, fomented by the then president of the United States, Donald Trump, took place in Washington, DC, during which the Capitol of the United States, the seat of the legislative bodies in the process of certifying the election of Joseph Biden, was invaded and desecrated, with blood and faeces smeared on walls and floors. Five deaths ensued, including one of the defenders of the Capitol, a policeman. The invaders in and beyond the Capitol carried flags: the battle flag of the Confederacy, the Gadsen 'Don't Tread on Me' Revolutionary War flag, both now signs of the far right, the American flag and the flag of Israel.[27] In the crowd Haredi Jews mixed with individuals wearing 'Camp Auschwitz: Work brings freedom' sweatshirts parodying the inscription at the gates of Auschwitz as well as other Nazi concentration and death camps.[28] As Jonathan Sarna, professor of American Jewish History at Brandeis University, noted, there were yet others whose 'T-shirt was emblazoned with the inscription "6MWE" above yellow symbols of Italian Fascism. "6MWE" is an acronym common among the far right standing for "6 Million Wasn't Enough." It refers to the Jews exterminated during the Nazi Holocaust and hints at the desire of the wearer to increase that number still further.'[29]

A number of ultra-Orthodox leaders of the anti-public health riots were involved in planning this, such as Heshy Tischler, who had helped organize the groups that invaded the Capitol, bussing them in from New York. He commented at the time that 'We want to be there . . . We just can't get in.' That Wednesday evening, after the mob had been allowed to leave the building, he opined, 'If I was actually in the front, I wouldn't have stormed, I would have walked in the doors.'[30] Visible in the crowd before the Capitol were numerous ultra-Orthodox Jews. Some of them were actually rioting inside the building. Thus Aaron Mostofsky entered the building wearing fur pelts and a bulletproof vest and carrying a stolen police riot shield. He and his brother Nachman, the executive director of Chovevei Zion, a politically conservative Orthodox advocacy organization that had organized a busload of demonstrators, were visible and active participants in the rally. Nachman was also a Brooklyn district leader and vice president of the South Brooklyn Conservative Club. They had come down from New York at the behest of the president, who promised in his tweet a few days earlier that 'it was going to be wild.'[31] Aaron was arrested by the FBI on 12 January and charged with unlawful entry of a restricted building and disorderly conduct on Capitol grounds with intent to impede government activity. He was charged with stealing the shield. His father, Kings County Supreme Court Judge Steven (Shlomo) Mostofsky, was the former president of the National Council of Young Israel, an Orthodox synagogue association that has been outspokenly pro-Trump. It was also one of the groups that most strongly objected to the public health measures, as

> singling out the Jewish community and its institutions is a form of discrimination that puts us at risk of a backlash from the broader population and unnecessarily fans the flames of the growing anti-Semitic sentiment that currently exists in the United States today. Houses of worship are a central part of Jewish communal life and inhibiting our ability to pray in our synagogues while simultaneously permitting gatherings to take place in other settings is an infringement of our First Amendment rights. By painting the Jewish community in a negative light while seemingly ignoring serious issues that exist in other areas and other communities during this pandemic, Governor Cuomo and Mayor de Blasio have employed a double standard when it comes to Orthodox Jews and synagogues that is discriminatory and dangerous. Synagogues and other houses of worship should be treated no differently from any other essential enterprise.[32]

This link of these communities with pro-Trump rhetoric as well as anti-public health rhetoric is not unexpected. One needs to remember that the Haredi community backed Trump overwhelmingly in 2016. As Elchanan Poupko, president of EITAN - The American Israeli Jewish Network, blogged in the *Times of Israel*, this community supported Trump, not specifically because of his so-called pro-Israel stance, but because of his anti-secular rhetoric. In the Hasidic New Square, 2,973 people cast their votes for Trump and 6 for Biden, and in the Satmar's Kiryas Joel 6,159 voted for Trump and just 72 for Biden.[33] Trump, whose rhetoric about the pandemic we shall discuss in greater detail in Chapter Five, came to be the symbol for a wide range of sentiments in the ultra-Orthodox community. While some of the Haredi organizations eventually issued statements abhorring the violence on that Wednesday, none condemned Trump's (and his followers') immediate and direct call for violence that touched off the invasion. Indeed, some of the leaders dismissed this attack on the state, as they had earlier dismissed attacks on the public health authorities. Yossi Gestetner, the head of the Orthodox Jewish Public Affairs Committee, tweeted to his followers to 'relax' and called the rioters' actions merely entering 'a building unauthorized'.[34] Pandemic denial as well as pandemic anxiety were also hallmarks of the Trump world image in 2020. Nothing much going on here, they seemed to say, just ignore the deaths, the blood and the horrors: you have had plenty of experience in doing this in your dealing with the pandemic.

The politics of the moment were clear as a community that had predominantly supported Donald Trump in 2016 and again in 2020 shouted his name over and over again at the demonstration. Trump represented a set of conservative values that the Haredi share with most evangelical Protestants (and conservative Catholics) and which centre on 'freedom of religion', which had come to be redefined as the 'first freedom' by Trump's executive order on 'Advancing International Religious Freedom' (2 June 2020). It has broadly redefined religious freedom to include state support for religious establishments of all types as well as the freedom of religious authorities from any interference in religious practice and belief, including attempts to mitigate the pandemic in these communities through specific limitations on the rates of occupancy in religious settings. Rabbi Yosef Blau, president of the Religious Zionists of America, explained this refocusing:

> Orthodox Jewry has become less concerned about the welfare of the broader society. The Trump administration was sympathetic to support for religious institutions. Political activity from Orthodox organizations in Washington is focused on increasing governmental response to Orthodox needs and supporting Israel. On issues facing the general society Orthodoxy has almost nothing to say.[35]

Perhaps the one major exception to this was the community's antipathy to public health interventions by state and local health authorities, at least in the case of the novel coronavirus.

That such antipathy could be quickly converted into a form of theological argument can be seen in the case of Gila Jedwab, a suburban New York 'maskless' dentist, who in her regular column in the local Jewish newspaper in June 2020 dismissed masking as ungodly:

> However, with this virus, when it came down to battling an unseen enemy, wouldn't the more intuitive approach be to let G-d handle this war without our help? We couldn't even see the enemy this time. Wouldn't it have been smarter to step aside and say, 'G-d, this battle is all You. We can't even see what we are fighting. Let's step back and let you handle it.' Trust does not look down on an entire world walking around in masks and say, 'good job.'[36]

Needless to say, she appeared without a mask during the 6 January 2021 'Save America' insurrection. The mask is otherwise neutral within Jewish ritual practice but because of the HIV/AIDS epidemic it became a requirement for dentists, who had been blamed for spreading the virus and who simultaneously saw themselves as at risk from their clients.

In Israel, Rabbi Chaim Kanievsky, the 93-year-old dean of the so-called Lithuanian Jews, a non-Hasidic sect of ultra-Orthodox Jews with Eastern European roots who form roughly a third of the Haredim in Israel, had also virulently opposed any closures of religious institutions, directly confronting state-mandated lockdowns, in spite of a massive spike of cases in his community. At the end of March 2020 the yeshivas (religious schools) were kept open in defiance of the first lockdown, and then were closed by the religious authorities, at least officially, with many students still surreptitiously holding classes and religious services. During the second lockdown in August/September 2020, the religious authorities defied the state and ordered them open. After Rosh Hashanah (New Year) celebrations more than 1,100 yeshiva students fell ill with the virus because of this flouting of state authority. Haim Zicherman, the academic director for the ultra-Orthodox campus of Ono Academic College, observed that this was 'the first time in the history of the state of Israel that the Haredim simply said, clearly and unequivocally, "We do not care what the law says; we are not going to obey."'[37] Soon, however, with a marked increase in morbidity and mortality, Kanievsky changed his views about the public's health. He advocated in June 2020 that wearing a mask, and in December that getting vaccinated, was a religious obligation.[38] His positions, however, were often so varied and contradictory that he became a litmus test for both acquiescence and objections to statemandated public health measures. Condemned earlier by secular society when he demanded that religious schools be kept open, his later advocacy of both masking and social distancing enabled his followers to pick and choose the symbols that seemed most relevant to them. Indeed, the mixed messages echoed the lobbying in the Haredi communities by Christian anti-vaxxing groups, who made the argument that such vaccinations represented bodily pollution against the will of God. As the medical anthropologist Ben Kasstan noted, the Haredi in 2020 'incorporate[d] [such] messages amidst evolving global–local encounters and via processes of discursive "conversion". Public criticism surrounding the ethics and safety of biomedical technologies circulates across physical and social borders, but also converts by undergoing a religious transformation of ideas and rationales.'[39] Thus the double binds that result are purposefully effective in selling an anti-state, anti-public health message that seems to have global cultural as well as local religious authority.

In the United States Rabbi Michoel Green, until January 2021 one of the official representatives for the Chabad (Lubavitch) movement, was fired from his position in Westborough, Massachusetts, as 'some of his public pronouncements were extremely reckless and potentially dangerous,' according to the regional leadership of Chabad. A fervent Trump supporter, Green publicly excoriated those who wore masks and obeyed social distancing guidelines. 'Lockdowns, widespread panic, masks, double masks, isolation, experimental gene therapy with lethal and reproductive risks, invasive but hardly diagnostic nasopharyngeal swabs and now anal swabs . . . All for a disease with a 99.9% survival rate.' When vaccines were made available, he stated, 'It's NOT immunization. It's pathogenic priming and mass sterilization.'[40] Being anti-mask became incorporated into an ultra-rightist vision of Jewish theology by being associated with the Trump right wing, even though the symbolic register of the right simultaneously included antisemitic conspiracy theories.

What such contradictions illustrate is that there is not a universal, continuous notion of the 'Jew'. Instead, each one of these parallel strands and their individual historical employment in the public sphere creates their own Jews who may or may not exist in the real world but who impact real people in the real world, including those who may or may not understand themselves as Jews, not because of theory but practice. Every antisemitic theory in its articulation in time and space invents its own Jews, and an awareness of that is vital if we are going to make any sense of 6 January 2021. The Haredi and indeed the Jews, however defined, who were at the Capitol knew that they were not the arch-Jewish villain George Soros and thus were quite comfortable being there. Whether the QAnon conspirators, waving their flag next to the Israeli flag, were happy with their presence is another, important question: each had invented its own Jews, for good or ill.

The symbolic register of 'Trump' during COVID-19 was also vital in redefining community boundaries within the United States, as ironically, given his role as head of the federal executive, he represented those who were anti-authoritarian, anti-science and, most importantly, anti-state control. Religion and state control were seen to be at odds. The legal exception even for those religious practices that refuse to employ allopathic medicine to treat ill co-religionists (and ultra-Orthodox Jews generally are not among them), such as Christian Science practitioners, has always had its limits in regard to infectious diseases. Mary Baker Eddy herself stated in 1902 that 'until public thought becomes better acquainted with Christian Science, the Christian Scientists shall decline to doctor infectious or contagious diseases.'[41]

Religion, certainly in the United States, has almost always had its practices limited, for good or for ill, when it has been perceived that these practices violate community standards (as in the case of the Indigenous use of peyote, which needed a Congressional exception in 1981 and then the passage of the American Indian Religious Freedom Act in 1994) or present a risk to the public's health beyond the bounds of the community. Thus, for example, the renewed contestation of the 'religious exception' to vaccination across a number of states with the spike in middle-class vaccine hesitancy in the early twenty-first century.

But the initial objections in the ultra-Orthodox community then were not to vaccination, although these did appear to a limited extent when vaccines were employed, but to non-pharmaceutical interventions such as social distancing, limitations on occupancy and masking. Earlier opposition to vaccines was based on the presence in some vaccines, such as those for measles (already contested in this as well as many Muslim communities), of porcine gelatine as a stabilizer. The first mRNA vaccines against the virus did not contain this. Naor Bar-Zeev, a professor of international health and vaccine science at the Johns Hopkins Bloomberg School of Public Health, noted that Jews were permitted to use xenographs as well as insulin from pigs: 'all these complex laws apply to food ingested by mouth and are not in any way relevant to injected material.'[42] Muslim religious authorities held much the same position. But the mRNA vaccines for COVID-19 did not present even this potential obstacle.

In Israel, as of April 2020, the ultra-Orthodox health minister Yaakov Litzman had refused to ban large religious meetings, until he too was diagnosed with the virus. When implemented, the global lockdown in Israel reduced the infection rate radically and by the end of the summer the restrictions were removed when ultra-Orthodox leaders rebelled against the further restriction of religious practice and the movement of thousands of religious students from abroad, primarily from New York City Orthodox communities, into Israel. In April 2020 New York City remained the epicentre of the infection, and the Orthodox community a particular focus for city health officials. The demands for isolation and distancing promulgated by Israel's newly appointed 'coronavirus czar', Dr Ronni Gamzu, were quickly undermined and he withdrew the most stringent of the controls when the ultra-Orthodox, who made up an important part of the government, began to attack the prime minister, Benjamin Netanyahu. 'The ultra-Orthodox point to the relative normalcy of life in Tel Aviv and complain that they are being singled out.'[43] The result was a radical spike in infection rates, to the point that Israel suddenly had one of the highest per capita rates in the world. In September the government again ordered another total closure to begin on the holiest week of the year, the Jewish New Year. The lockdown triggered an immediate response – it was read as an attack on religious believers. Yaakov Litzman, now the minister of housing and construction, resigned his portfolio. He was 'furious that the restrictions would coincide with Rosh Hashana and Yom Kippur, the annual day of fasting and atonement, and that worshipers would be allowed in synagogues only in limited numbers. He said the government had delayed acting earlier for fear of spoiling Israelis' summer vacation plans.'[44] What Litzman did was to identify the source of blame, the state, as motivated by 'Jewish' antisemitism. In his opinion, the public health authorities were not attempting to control major sources of the outbreak but rather using this claim as an ideological weapon aimed at Haredim by the majority of secular Jews. (Not that he was wrong: the condemnations of the Haredi communities were widespread among secular groups in Israel, while they themselves crowded Tel-Aviv's beaches, held large public demonstrations against the government and attended house parties as surreptitious as the learning in the closed yeshivas.) Litzman was echoing the April 2020 attacks on the police and health authorities in Mea Sharim, the ultra-Orthodox neighbourhood of Jerusalem, which labelled these forces as well as the then minister of health – Litzman himself – as 'Nazis'.[45]

During the third lockdown in Israel, the Netanyahu-dominated coalition government, facing a fourth election since April 2019, showed amazing competence in its ability to vaccinate the largest proportion of its citizenry of any nation-state, given the global limitations on the availability of the vaccines.[46] Yet it also demonstrated incompetence concerning public health measures as local opposition to masking and social distancing continued. While they make up 12.8 per cent of the Israeli population, ultra-Orthodox communities came to have 28 per cent of the cases by the end of the year. In late January 2021 riots broke out in ultra-Orthodox neighbourhoods in Jerusalem. In Bnei Brak the rioters belonged to an extremist faction of the Vizhnitz Hasidic sect, but were joined by many others on the street. A bus was fire-bombed, police cars burned and police who responded attacked. They in turn responded with water cannon and stun grenades. The government did little or nothing to ameliorate these civil insurrections, having already diminished the ability of the public health authorities to deal with the extraordinary extent of the out-break again in these communities, because of the government's reliance on the religious parties for electoral support.

COVID-19 has forced a reckoning with what had been an ongoing shift within the ultra-Orthodox world. As with African American women, as we shall discuss in Chapter Four, Haredi women have joined the workforce in ever-growing numbers over the past decade. Haredi men, especially young men, have begun to sense shifts in the symbolic order of their world. The effect of such shifts in Israel was exacerbated as the progress towards total vaccination of the entire population in early 2021 seemed to be thwarted, over and over again, by ultra-Orthodox activities, from anti-lockdown riots to mass funerals. As one middle-aged ultra-Orthodox woman in Bnei Brak, Vivian Shinfeld, noted, 'Now it's not only tense – it feels like hatred. Now it is starting to feel like a war.' Her husband added, 'If the government says, "Wear a mask," that's a reason for them not to wear a mask.'[47] Anti-vaccination attitudes were grounded in a mistrust of the state by these communities, a state, however, in which their political parties have a prominent role. Posters appeared in their neighbourhoods reading 'Jews, open your eyes, why rush? The gentiles can get vaccinated first.'[48] And indeed, although Israel by late February 2021 had the highest per capita rate of vaccination of any nation-state, these communities lagged substantially. Vaccination hesitancy is a political position.

Conflict between secular (including non-Haredi religious) Israelis and what come more and more to be perceived as anti-state forces within a world in which the ultra-Orthodox have real political power, as in the Israeli government in 2020, parallels the position of American ultra-Orthodox Jews in the world of Trump, where their votes helped elect him in 2016 and where he continued to stress their ongoing importance. The confusion of symbolic regimes in a world with shifting value systems and the radical defence of them is the sort of double bind that demands a resolution – yet this is impossible to achieve.

After Rabbi Meshulam Soloveitchik, the head of the Brisk Yeshiva (religious school) in Jerusalem, died of the virus in late

January 2021 at the age of 99, over 20,000 mainly unmasked mourners accompanied the coffin.[49] Again, the police were stymied, even though Benny Gantz, speaking for the opposition, saw such activities as making a mockery of the lockdown. One-tenth of the Israeli population are ultra-Orthodox but in January 2021 they recorded one-third of the infections nationwide. The religious authorities, including the now housing minister Yaakov Litzman, simply laid the violence at the feet of the police. The analogy was, of course, to the Holocaust: a resident of one of the neighbourhoods, Nathan Rosenblatt, spoke about 'the *Kristallnacht* that the police carried out in Bnei Brak last week'. A representative of the extremist Jerusalem Faction accused police of carrying out 'pogroms'.[50] In the Knesset, the deputy speaker for one of the ultra-Orthodox parties, Israel Eichler, condemned the restrictions on Haredi neighbourhoods – 'as if they were ghettos' – and claimed that the secular state, at least in terms of its public health mandates, was antisemitic, as well as that to say the Hasidim were to blame for spreading the virus was 'a racist defamation, as if they are the disseminators of disease and contamination', which 'engenders anti-Semitism among a population fearful of the virus all over the country'.[51] Jews blaming Jews is a form of Nazi behaviour, even if such claims were actually valid both in raw numbers as well as in the lived experience of those in the ultra-Orthodox communities.

The power of the instrumentalization of history is clearest during the reaction to the public health measures taken to ameliorate COVID-19. Given the projection of such images of the Holocaust and the 'SS State' onto contemporary state public health actors, both in the United States and Israel, the arrogation in Germany among the followers of the nationalist and far-right political party Alternative für Deutschland of yellow mock 'Jewish star' armbands with the word 'Ungeimpft' (unvaccinated) seems apposite.[52] Indeed, the evocation of the Holocaust became a set trope for the opponents of virtually every public health measure, from wearing masks to the closing of public spaces, not only in Germany but across the Western world. As the Holocaust had become the historical moment that defined 'victimhood', even those engaged in antisemitic conspiracy theories concerning the Rothschilds and the 'International Jewish Conspiracy' appropriated these symbols.

Suddenly, every player, ultra-Orthodox Jew or not, becomes the metaphoric victim of state power, of the Nazis. In Britain the anti-state actors, calling themselves 'StandUp X', went even further. Online they state that their membership 'does not consent to the "illegal and disproportionate measures"' and argues that Britain is 'living in a state of authoritarian control. Social distancing measures, the wearing of masks, the enforcement of lockdowns and "Covid Ghettos" are among the rules and regulations StandUp X opposes.' They make the argument that the use of vaccines, especially, turns them into subjects of medical experiments that 'violate the principles of the Nuremberg Code'.[53] Not merely victims, but victims of the Nazis, forced into ghettos and subject to horrific medical violations.

COVID Redivivus

At the close of 2020 the spike in the number of cases in Israel to 5,000 a day led to a third partial national shutdown. By 1 January 2021, 420,000 Israelis had been infected and 3,325 had died. The focus by this point was no longer on the Haredi and Israeli Arab communities as being more at risk than the general population and as a greater threat for transmitting the virus. What became a national focus after 20 December 2020 was mass vaccination. With a rigorously organized system of interlocking community health structures, to which all citizens belonged, able to deliver vaccines and a government that early on arranged to purchase them, by the beginning of the year, Israel saw almost 10 per cent of its population having received the first dose of the available mRNA vaccines, better than almost any other nation on earth. The minister of health in the so-called unity government, Yuli Edelstein, saw mass vaccination as not only a public health necessity but a chance to use the health system as a basis for further testing and research on the efficaciousness of the vaccines. Israel, including most of its inhabitants, would become a laboratory to measure the efficacy of the vaccines. (The question of access, specifically to the Palestinian occupants of the 'occupied territories' on the West Bank and Gaza, presented another, major public health challenge, as unvaccinated workers from the West Bank did cross into the state on a daily basis. It was only in March 2021 that this population began to receive inoculations.) On 19 December 2020 the prime minister, Benjamin Netanyahu, was the first person in Israel to be publicly vaccinated. He stated, 'We brought [the vaccines] to everyone: Jews and Arabs, religious and secular.'[54] The ultra-religious, fractured over the issue of state controls of the public's health, did not see this as analogous to social control. Rabbi Yitzchok Zilberstein, a leading ultra-Orthodox authority (posek) in Jewish medical ethics and the rabbi of the Ramat Elchanan neighbourhood of Bnei Brak, advocated strongly for the vaccine, noting that the vaccine 'should be taken even by healthy people based on the imperative of "Ve'Rapo Ye'Rapeh", which requires taking medicines even if there is some risk'.[55] This supports medical anthropologist Ben Kasstan's earlier observation that Haredi rabbinic authorities in Israel generally advocate for vaccination and that even if there were to be anti-vaxxers who saw this as state overreach, this would not be the official religious view.[56] Yet the conflict of such views with the symbolic regime of global anti-vaxxers, which held vaccination in the same register as masking and lockdowns, meant that these communities had a consistently lower rate of vaccination when vaccines became available.

Yet the third wave continued to impact the ultra-Orthodox communities well out of proportion to all other communities in Israel. Within the four weeks from the beginning of December 2020 to early January 2021, their rate of infection increased sixteenfold. By 7 January 2021 the mutant variant initially discovered in Britain was raging in the ultra-Orthodox community, accounting for more than 20 per cent of its morbidity. While earlier flaunting of requirements for masking, social distancing and limitations on crowd size had been ignored by many within these communities, the new spike, which amounted to over 4,000 cases a day (in a population of about 9 million) by the end of February 2021, as predicted by Eran Segal of the Weizmann Institute of Science, may well have had yet a further cause.[57] We need to imagine that such ideologically and physically interlaced communities, in Britain, the United States and Israel, have seen community spread exactly because of the so-called 'insularity' of these communities and their regular commerce with one with another.

Let us now think about the construction of blame and its historicization within self-defined communities, large and small, in such a context. Self-defined communities are constituted by elective isolation from the greater society, by systematic isolation by the greater society, by ghettoization, a complex term, as Daniel B. Schwartz has noted, that starts with Venetian Jews in

1516 and comes to encompass the spaces inhabited by margin-alized peoples from Jim Crow America, to Chinatowns across the world, to the Nazi arenas of forced isolation and death, to those occupied by refugees in contemporary Europe.[58] Through all these the image of the ghetto was connected to infectious diseases caused by its inhabitants; as Schwartz notes, the ghetto was 'a site of material filth and disorder' already by the six-teenth century.[59] Yet, as Schwartz observes, the concept was repatriated by American Jews, who were as much focused on hygiene as they were on acculturation. Writers such as Abraham Cahan, in his *Yekl: A Tale of the New York Ghetto* (1896), saw these clearly defined spaces as functioning as 'an assimilative "melting pot".'[60] Many Jews in the American diaspora saw the ghetto as a 'constitutive element of Jewish identity'.[61] After the Second World War it became for other Jews 'a metaphor for a premodern Jewish past destined for obliteration, but one that survived as a spectral presence'.[62] Urban sociologists saw this in equally complex ways, removing the ghetto from the world of disease to one of caste. The Chicago School, under Robert E. Park, moved the ghetto as a space of disjuncture to an imagined community, as in Louis Wirth's classic *The Ghetto* (1928), which transformed the ghetto from 'a Jewish site to a sociological con-cept'.[63] Indeed, it had already become part of the standard way in which concentrated zones of social habitation were mapped by Park's colleague Ernest W. Burgess in 1925. Yet the negative connotations of ill health, filth and disorder seem to be pres-ent even in these 'scientific' contexts, as one can see in Daniel Patrick Moynihan's infamous 1965 account of the breakdown of the 'Negro family' in the ghetto.[64] Communities can be ghettos, and those living within their real or symbolic space respond to these metaphoric constructions of the health dangers within by becoming hyperaware of the stigma associated with them. All are part then of the complex symbolic register used by those self-defined as victims of state authority in the COVID-19 crisis.

The public's health or the new Nazis? Antisemitism or a reasonable, measured response? Some people or all people? Here is the problem that we face: can you discuss pandemics without stereotypes being evoked as either a weapon against specific groups or a defence for these groups? How do we see the categories that emerge in defining populations in the discourse of public health as separate from or part of such analysis?

Explanations for Placing the Blame

Let us look at a series of interlocking problems that lurk behind the assumptions concerning the placing of blame on ultra-Orthodoxy. The rationales provided for the explosion of infections in ultra-Orthodox communities in the United States and Israel must begin by first defining what and where such communities are and how they define themselves, and second, based on these definitions, trying to imagine how the core problem can be situated in the intersection between religious communities and state power, such as in concerns for the public's health.

The general discourse about the pandemic lumps all ultra-Orthodox communities and their members together and labels them as Haredim. In fact, these groups cover a very wide range of ideological positions, including those concerning the public's health. On the margin are the radical anti-Zionist and isolationist Haredim such as Neturei Karta, a religious group formally created in Jerusalem in 1938, who sponsored crowded and unmasked marches against the State of Israel in Jerusalem in late November 2020. When the earlier outbreak occurred in the spring in Mea

Shearim, the Jerusalem neighbourhood where the majority of the Neturei Karta dwell, the admonition was to 'follow the Torah'. 'Our rabbi said to continue praying.'[65] The twelve Hasidic rabbinic 'courts' too are diverse, from the highly political Ger (the largest community in Israel), to the Satmar and Bobov (the largest in New York City) communities led by inherited rabbinic leadership, to the global group the Lubavitchers (known worldwide under the name Chabad), whose absence of leadership and desire for the resurrection of their late rabbi Menachem Mendel Schneerson (who died in 1994) has led the sociologists Menachem Friedman and Samuel Heilman to see them as more closely aligned to Messianic Christianity awaiting a Second Coming than main-stream ultra-Orthodox Jewry.[66] In Israel (as with their Trump Republican orientation in the United States) many of these ultra-Orthodox groups align with specific political parties that have a wide range of opinions about the public's health. Agudath Israel (now the central organization of Haredi Jews in the United States) in Borough Park, Brooklyn, for example, distributed more than half a million masks, while in the same community cele-brations for Sukkot in 2020 brought together large numbers of unmasked worshippers for massive indoor services.[67] The official organization advocated for adherence to public health guide-lines. 'Simchos (*sic*) [celebrations] that spread illness and do not conform to local laws should not be allowed to jeopardize . . . a return to a sense of normalcy.'[68] Yet such actions by some come to characterize the community in its totality. As Yehuda Meshi-Zahav, the head of ZAKA, Israel's voluntary emergency response organization, noted in October 2020,

> I explain to people that others are looking at them, and saying that we're in this situation because of Haredim, and

that the 12 percent is infecting the 80-plus percent, and that 'you' are 'stealing' the breathing machines. And I say that this hatred is terrible, but what people see is the continuation of singing, dancing, public prayers, and simchas [celebrations] – as well as continuation of protests. If Jews are saying the things . . . about each other, of course others will say them . . . They will take the symbol of a man in Jewish dress, and connect it to the coronavirus.[69]

Haredi Jews, he notes, in Israel and in the diaspora, by their actions come to represent all Jews.

In the United Kingdom the largest ultra-Orthodox communities are in London, Essex (with new ultra-Orthodox communities at Southend-on-Sea) and Manchester and consist of a wide range of groups aligned with the national Union of Orthodox Hebrew Congregations. All these groups have taken often contradictory positions, some articulated by their rabbinic leadership, some by members (often in positions of political power) and some by lay leaders. These positions have varied from complete support of all public health measures to combat the pandemic, to total rejection, back to modified acceptance of certain limitations at certain times and in certain contexts. There have also been radical realignments of such positions over time. As Nadav Davidovitch, director of the School of Public Health at Ben-Gurion University of the Negev, states, 'the haredi community is not monolithic; it has many parts . . . Some of them have very good compliance [rates]. Some of them [at the same time] have a long history of defying the Zionist state.'[70] This is equally true in the United States and the United Kingdom. The key in the UK as well as in Israel and in the United States is the conceptual structure of 'community'. A recent court case in London, focused on whether Agudat Israel, the Orthodox community charity, could limit occupation of its housing units to religious Jews, was won by the community. Rabbi Abraham Pinter, who was to die of COVID-19 in April 2020, stressed in his testimony that 'being part of a community, both physically and spiritually, is a prerequisite of fulfilling the life of an Orthodox Jew.'[71] What the term 'community' means is central to any understanding of discussions about infection and group responses.

If the ultra-Orthodox community is not homogenous in its construction, it does also not simply consist of large families living on the edge of poverty. This rationale has been regularly provided to explain the much higher rates of transmission in these communities. When the first major outbreak took place in suburban Ultra-Orthodox communities in Rockland County, the local rabbi Yisroel Kahanin attributed the higher rate of infection in the spring of 2020 to such circumstances:

> In communities where people have larger families, and with Passover coming, people wanted to get tested to know whether they had it and whether they were safe to be at grandma's and watch over them . . . Once those numbers were out there and it looked like Monsey was on the high end of the county, where Monsey is now on the lower end, you had the haters coming out of the woodwork.[72]

An editorial in the *Jerusalem Post* in April stressed 'poverty and the challenge of confining large families in small apartments' as 'the main things to blame'.[73] Yet there are clearly middle-class religious Jews in such communities in the United States and Israel whose living environment is very different from and whose rate of infection is similar to their poorer religious compatriots.

The poverty and resultant crowded living conditions of the Haredim in Israel and the United States are argued to be causal for community spread. Certainly, individual income (at least in 2013) of ultra-Orthodox Jews in the United States was lower than that of other Jews (43 per cent of the former and 37 per cent of the latter earned below $50,000). But one needs to note that 24 per cent of Haredim in 2013 had incomes in excess of $150,000, higher than Conservative Jews (23 per cent) and substantially higher than the general American public (8 per cent). While the poverty rate was attributable to a lower level of secular education (25 per cent have a college education as compared to 58 per cent of all Jews and 29 per cent of the overall American population), no comment is made about the upper end of the economic scale.[74] But what secular education means in this community is quite different and such poverty is offset by state support from SNAP to Medicaid. One can add that such figures examine individual income, not the potential wealth of the collective community, augmented by the role that charity played supported by the higher earners in it. In Israel, while the overall income rates are lower, with 58 per cent of Haredi families living below the official poverty line in 2018, the shifts in family earning capacity over the past decade and ever stronger state economic support make these communities content with their economic status. Only 8 per cent felt that they were living in poverty, while 71 per cent were satisfied with the economic situation. Thus at a time where secular Israeli society was up in arms about economic pressures, two-thirds felt they were economically disadvantaged. The reality in Israel was that because of state and community support many fewer ultra-Orthodox reported food insufficiencies (10 per cent) than Israeli Arabs (14 per cent).[75] Poverty is also part of a symbolic system; if you understand yourself as 'poor', you see yourself as excluded rather than included in the community.

Sociability rather than poverty is at the core of some readings of the radical increases in infection rates, a sociability defined by the very construction of the symbolic language of the community. Shaul Magid, professor of Jewish Studies at Dartmouth, and formerly a member of such a community, noted in a personal message that

> the haredi community is a much more social community than most of us live in. By social I mean that the collective life is driven by social events, from as small as daily minyan, night *seder*, to as big as a *hasidishe* wedding or the rebbe's table on *Sukkos*. These events don't have the same values in our world as in theirs. For them, this is the crux of their 'leisure' time, it is largely where people meet outside business or study. I recall being surprised when I entered the haredi world that children were always a part of that social world. The notion of children not being invited to weddings is unheard of.[76]

But at the same time child abuse, isolation and alienation are present in these communities, as in all communities.[77] From the novels of Chaim Potok in the 1960s to the 2020 television series *Unorthodox*, these themes have become a standard part of mass culture. The pandemic in Israel has also led to a radical increase of those leaving the community in reality rather than fiction. While about 3,000 Haredim left yearly over the past decade, this number spiked by over 50 per cent over the course of 2020. The simple exposure to the debates about the pernicious social isolation of the community and its responsibility for the spread of the pandemic was evidently a factor. Gilad Malach, of the Israel Democracy Institute, noted that with the loosening of the structures of the community, at which Magid gestured, because of the pandemic, 'They think of options they don't think of when they are in yeshiva, and one of the options is to leave.'[78] And leave they do, in spite of the powerful drive to conform to the community's norms and the comfort of their known symbolic world.

The other take on the uniform nature of such communities is that it is the religious leadership that is able to manipulate their followers into destructive acts. Bad, ineffectual leadership of cowed communities without resources leads to the spread of the disease. No one articulated this with more vigour than Yitz Greenberg, the Modern Orthodox rabbi and founder, chairman and professor in the department of Jewish studies of the City College of New York, when he wrote in the *Jerusalem Post* that:

> by and large the religious leadership has been a drag on the efforts to contain the pandemic. Where it has not outright encouraged policies that increased transmission, it often posed obstacles to needed actions. Rabbis both haredi (ultra-Orthodox) and hardal (nationalist haredi), insisted that the yeshivot learning Torah should go on even though they were spreading the virus . . . The outcome is that haredi and traditional religious communities have the highest rates of infection, other than Arabs, and disproportionate numbers of deaths and serious cases with damaging after effects.[79]

While explaining who is at fault, such arguments tend to lump all ultra-Orthodox communities in Israel (and by extension elsewhere) together as inherently corrupt because of the very nature of how the communities are constituted.

The condemnation of all rabbinic authorities in Israel was answered in a blistering editorial by Rabbi Avi Shafran, the director of public affairs of Agudat Israel, in the same newspaper, claiming that it was the situation of the neighbourhoods, not their leadership, that was to blame.

> No, it wasn't because of the density of many haredi towns and neighborhoods. Nor were the regular interactions born of religious events, celebrations, and daily prayer services salient factors. And no, poverty, and the challenge of confining large families in small apartments were not the main things to blame. Jewish religious leaders, Rabbi Greenberg contends, are viewed by haredim as infallible. This is nonsense. The reason Jewish religious leaders are respected is their sensitivity and Torah scholarship, and that is very different from blind obedience.[80]

There are certainly other, more impoverished non-religious communities in Israel, for example Ethiopian (Beta Israel) neighbourhoods in Netanya, Beersheva and Ashdod, which have suffered from COVID-19, but where the community leadership was more proactive or at least not obstructionist. Indeed, immigration from Ethiopia was put on hold during the pandemic at a time when American and European yeshiva students were allowed into the country and reopened only on 12 October 2020, but with much-reduced numbers.[81] The yeshiva students were admitted because of the intercession of rabbinic authorities (and their concomitant political representatives); the Ethiopian refugees had no such representations to speak for them in the chambers of power.

If we acknowledge that transmission is certainly enhanced by poor living conditions and encouragement to ignore voluntary or even required quarantine measures, we are still left with the question of why these particular out-groups, in all their diversity, are seen as a major source of infection, when many other analogous groups, with equally high or indeed higher infection rates, are not. Yossi Gestetner, co-founder of the Orthodox Jewish Public Affairs Council in New York, opined:

> When there [are] disproportionate numbers of African-American deaths because of corona, there isn't one reporter in any outlet that suggests that anything is wrong with African-Americans as a community because of their behavior . . . It's about disparities, institutional racism, and poverty; which is fine because the idea to take people who are victimized [by] a problem and make [the problem] about them is unheard of bigotry.[82]

The charge of antisemitism refocused attention on what was labelled as the conditions of transmission, including poverty and overcrowding. The implications were that these conditions were the direct result of the systemic antisemitism under which Jews lived in the United States or Israel rather than a reflection of the values of the community that held religious study above secular gains. This accounts for radically different values attributed to concepts such as poverty and leadership. These actions were defined by the sense that such communities abided by a different set of symbols than the secular world. We need to note here that, especially in the United States, the extraordinarily higher rate of infection present among people of colour has also been explained by poverty, which results in poor and crowded living conditions, but this is a reflection of the systemic racism in American society imposed on these communities.[83] One can add to these effects by tabulating other products of caste that were causal in the higher rates of morbidity and mortality in this community: subsistence or 'essential' occupations (garbage collectors, shop attendants, workers in slaughterhouses, health-care personnel) and pre-existing health conditions, including mental health, directly caused by marginalization and displace-ment all played a role. This seems to be equally true in the UK, where hospitalization and death rates among Black, Asian and minority ethnic (BAME) communities were higher than those of White British people. This appears to be due to a complex mixture of factors, and no one factor alone can explain all the differences. Contributing factors include, in no particular order: 'being poorer, where people live, overcrowded housing, types of job, other illnesses, and access to health services.'[84] Why, Jewish commentators ask, is it possible to condemn Haredi commun-ities living in analogous circumstances while giving communities of colour not only a pass, but empathy for their situation?

That poverty and race are seen as coterminous is generally true, but this is no more uniform in these communities of colour than in the Haredi world. The economic status of Black women in the United States and the United Kingdom, for example, has been ever-increasing over the past decades. It is clear that such communities may well not be called out as sources of infection because of anxieties about labelling using race in an age of Black Lives Matter (BLM). Yet, as we shall see in Chapter Four of this study, such communities contain the core of identical contra-dictions, shaped not as much by history and memory as they are by their evocation in 2020. One can note that self-defined communities, which in point of fact exist both as a response to social segregation and voluntary separation, in both national states, may look similar but their lived experiences may be very different. The real question in all cases is the limitation on individual agency and the resonance of state mandates as guidelines to action within these communities.

If negative images of resistance to state authority are seen as part of ultra-Orthodoxy's response to the pandemic, it is equally true that there is also an assumption of the specific nature of resilience in such self-contained communities. In London's ultra-Orthodox community in Stamford Hill, according to *The Guardian*,

> The virus has shone a light on cracks in every community, but it has also unearthed resilience. The close-knit way of life in Stamford Hill meant lockdown presented previously unimaginable challenges and many were at risk. Everybody knows people who have died. Equally, those . . . who needed support in a moment of need have undoubtedly received it. Moses Gluck, the undertaker, echoed so many I spoke to when he told me his work was not just business; 'there has to be heart to it'.[85]

In January 2021 Stamford Hill, which is part of the borough of Hackney, had a COVID-19 infection rate of 625.43 cases per 100,000 people. The average rate in England in January 2021 was 471.31 per 100,000 people. Yet resistance continued during the third British lockdown, as a wedding with more than four hundred participants crowded into Yesodey Hatorah Senior Girls' School in Stamford Hill in early January 2021. The school's headmaster, Avrahom Pinter, had died of COVID-19 in April 2020. The participants fled when the police entered the building. The Chief

(Orthodox) Rabbi of the UK and Commonwealth Ephraim Mirvis condemned the action as 'a most shameful desecration of all that we hold dear. At a time when we are all making such great sacrifices, it amounts to a brazen abrogation of the responsibility to protect life and such illegal behaviour is abhorred by the overwhelming majority of the Jewish community.'[86] Evidently such weddings had continued *sub rosa* during the entirety of 2020, with multiple weddings per day with many hundreds of guests taking place at a large series of venues throughout Stamford Hill. There was little enforcement of the various lockdowns and no policing of the documented spread of the virus to participants and service personnel. A leading member of the ultra-Orthodox community simply gave up on any notion of social responsibility for the increased spread: 'Trying to explain, justify or mitigate [the large weddings] doesn't work. People feel too strongly about it. No one is going to back down. It has already generated an unprecedented amount of negative coverage of the Stamford Hill community, in some cases well-deserved. But it is what it is.' They are not us, says a representative of the non-Orthodox community: 'It lets the side down. Not only that, it's downright dangerous. Yes, it is important not to stigmatise a whole community . . . We don't hold Jewish weddings at certain times of the year because of a plague that happened 2,000 years ago, yet the plague we're living through now doesn't appear reason enough to postpone.'[87] Was this resistance, resilience or rebellion?

In Israel the confrontation with state authority during the second lockdown in October 2020 was seen by some in terms of alternative forms of resistance and resilience. The Israeli government has defined itself as 'Jewish' since the passage of the new nation-state 'nationality Law' in 2018. It was no longer 'the nation state for the Jewish people' as stated in the 1950 Basic

Law, which had also recognized Israeli Arab citizens as having equal legal and cultural status. This expressly 'Jewish' government, headed by the prime minister, Benjamin Netanhayu, who advocated and passed the 2018 law, locked down the nation for a second time on 17 October 2020, and thus came to be defined as the enemy. This led to a form of resistance among some ultra-Orthodox Jews in Mea Sharim, an ultra-Orthodox section of Jerusalem, who refused to test symptomatic people through state public health mechanisms, turning rather to a private charity, Hasdei Amram, to deal with their treatment and isolation. The ministry of health denounced such measures, labelling them as dangerous and most probably illegal, since the infections were not reported to the state and adherence to quarantine rules could not be monitored.[88] Resistance and resilience as seen from beyond and within such communities differ widely and are interpreted accordingly.

Imagined Nations

During the Enlightenment there was increased reliance on a specific code of symbols, forcing such a 'state within a state' and 'nation within a nation' as the Jews, here citing Hannah Arendt's discussion of the origins of antisemitism, to accommodate Jewish public life to the national symbolic register. For, as Arendt further observed, while the 'Jews had no political ambitions of their own and were merely the only social group that was unconditionally loyal to the state, [the antisemites] were half right . . . because the Jews, taken as a social and not as a political body, actually did form a separate group within the nation.'[89] Such a desire for radical integration into the nation-state can call forth from within such subsumed communities a defensive posture reflecting a heightened community autonomy. Some German Jews, as Arendt notes, were quite happy in general to abandon their parochial identity for a new national identity, meaning a new symbolic register for their sense of community, perhaps more than any other group in the new Germany.[90] But there was resistance even within the various Jewish communities in what would become Germany after 1871. The symbolic register of nationalism that some German Jews adopted was an idealistic German nationalism, as espoused in the Enlightenment by figures such as J. G. Herder and Friedrich Schiller, which contained more than a little antisemitic rhetoric. The argument, most clearly stated in revolutionary France by Comte de Clermont-Tonnerre in 1789, was that civil rights could be granted to any individual (Jew) but not to the Jews as a 'nation'. Modern Orthodox thinkers rebelled against these forms of identification that vitiated community boundaries.

Yet one needs to understand the centrality of the public sphere in modernity. One of its core concepts that helps shape such positions is the political rebranding of religious communities as bounded political entities in the light of Lockean notions of citizenship's relationship to religious practice. This is the complex problem that one finds in nation-states where some groups of Jews do not subsume their political symbolic identity to that of the state. Indeed, recently, with the second outbreak of COVID-19 in Israel and their renewed resistance to state public health authority, the ultra-Orthodox community have been dismissed by Gilad Malach at an independent think tank, who calls them 'a state within a state' that places the entire nation-state at risk, for 'if 50% of the sick are Haredim, it affects the whole country.'[91] Thus the ultra-Orthodox are the 'Jews' within the 'antisemitic' Israeli state (now officially defined as 'Jewish'), a conundrum only explainable through the rejection of conflicting symbolic identification with a single 'imagined community', as already discussed by Hannah Arendt as the goal of Enlightenment integration. In this reading Israel becomes Germany after 1933; the ultra-Orthodox, the secular and religious Jews of Berlin and Frankfurt under the Nuremburg Laws.

John Locke's 1689 'Letter Concerning Toleration' aimed its barbs at the Hobbesian notion that homogeneity in religion was a necessary prerequisite for a functioning state. (We shall discuss Hobbes in more detail in Chapter Five.) Identification with a powerful symbolic system such as religion could only undermine any identification with the totality of the state. Locke not only advocated pluralism but demanded a border between religious belief and state function, to 'distinguish exactly the business of civil government from that of religion and to settle the just bounds that lie between the one and the other. If this be not done, there can be no end put to the controversies that will be always arising between those that have, or at least pretend to have, on the one side, a concernment for the interest of men's souls, and, on the other side, a care of the commonwealth.'[92] While anxious about extending Catholics civil rights in Great Britain, he imagined these rights being extended if the Roman Church abdicated its claims to civil authority. Religious belief has its boundaries in the secular state, which cannot regulate the soul; the secular state's civil powers, however, were universal over the citizen's actions, not the citizen's beliefs. The key was the demand that each religion tolerate the state's authority and that the state tolerate a diversity of religious views (excluding, of course, atheism – even Locke would not have tolerated that).

Within the Enlightenment tradition, Jewish reformers, following Moses Mendelssohn, made the distinction between religious practice within the community and civil actions in the greater society. Here they followed the classic definition of the Enlightenment stated by Immanuel Kant, who, however, was loath to include the Jews (at least the Polish Jews) in a world in which the individual was able to abandon the 'the guidance of another', having the 'lack of the resolution and the courage to use it without the guidance of another. *Sapere aude!* Have the courage to use your own understanding! is thus the motto of enlightenment!'[93] The Jews saw this as a call to re-examine the assumptions not only of religious practice but of the very notion of the symbolic language of their 'imagined community', in Benedict Anderson's sense, as we discussed in Chapter One. As Jonathan A. Jacobs notes, as a result of these shifts, 'many Jews have chosen not to accept the responsibility to fulfill the commandments . . . while still identifying strongly as Jews, as members of the Jewish people, committed to democratic values.'[94] Such an identification with the symbolic vocabulary of the post-Enlightenment nation-state may also drive other Jews, more strongly identifying with their existing 'imagined' religious community, to be conflicted between its existing symbolic definition and that of the new public sphere, which, as Jacobs correctly argues, demands a certain neutrality vis-à-vis what we have come to call the symbolic register of the state.

Such a re-examination necessarily led, as Antoon Braeckman notes, to 'the plea for the emancipation of thinking' but also to modifications of religious practice when such practice contradicted civil society's rules, rules that were also being formulated as 'manners' at the same moment for the rising bourgeoisie of all faiths during the Enlightenment.[95] Thus religious practice and civil society were mutually self-defining. Religious societies, such as Catholics, Jews and Muslims, which understood no boundary between civic society and religious practice were forced to choose between the two.[96] Some chose to remain isolated from secular society, as did the Church after the Risorgimento, at least after 1871, locking the gates of the Vatican until the Lateran treaty of 1929 between Pius XI and Mussolini's fascist government allowed the establishment of a new nation-state, Vatican City, with its own symbolic values. Jews in Western Europe approached such adaptation gingerly. Some reformed Jews advocated abandoning those practices, such as ritual slaughter of animals and infant male circumcision, that were anathema in (Christian) secular Europe. At the same time in Eastern Europe, the Haskalah, the Jewish Enlightenment, confronted not secularizing states but rigidly defined monarchies; indeed, after Catherine the Great refused to amend civil law in Russia following an Enlightenment model, the Jews there, very few of whom became Russified, remained in homogenous settlements socially and culturally isolated from their urban neighbours. Their boundaries were established by the state in 1791 through the so-called 'Pale of Settlement', where Jews were permitted to live, and by radical limitations on official Jewish residence in urban areas beyond the Pale. By the end of the nineteenth century a reaction to such radical acceptance of civil boundaries in the West led to modern Orthodoxy, with Samson Raphael Hirsch's evocation of the ancient trope of 'Torah im Derech Eretz' (Religion in the Context of the Nation-state), which more closely limited the relationship between observant Jews and secular society. For Hirsch in his *Religion Allied to Progress* (1854):

> Judaism is not a mere adjunct to life: it comprises all of
> life. To be a Jew is not a mere part, it is the sum total of our
> task in life. To be a Jew in the synagogue and the kitchen,

in the field and the warehouse, in the office and the pulpit . . . with the needle and the graving-tool, with the pen and the chisel – that is what it means to be a Jew.[97]

But he also stressed the need to acquire secular knowledge and to use such knowledge to function as a Jew in the greater world; there was to be no compromise of religious practice but some accommodation to secular demands, a clear answer to the Reformers' view of 'a Jew at home; a citizen on the street'. Hirsch's relationship to the first modern age of biological medicine can be seen in his statement that Jewish ritual practice concerning infectious diseases (such as Hansen's disease, then still known as leprosy) did not imply any hygiene enforcement by those 'officials in the service of . . . sanitation'.[98] For Hirsch acknowledges the fact that Jewish interpretation did not distinguish between a wide range of infectious 'diseases of the skin', from 'leprosy' to 'the diseases of modern Europe', such as measles and scarlet fever. In addition Jewish ritual law on the isolation of Jews with such diseases did not extend to those non-Jews in the same community. Religion and the public's health were to be two separate aspects of the symbolic register for modern Orthodoxy. It is of little surprise that Hirsch's granddaughter, Rahel Hirsch, became one of the first women physicians trained in the German-speaking world in 1903. For what today is seen as the bulwark of ultra-Orthodoxy, centred in the rabbinic courts of Eastern Europe, even modern Orthodoxy's moderate rapprochement to secular society was one step too far. For many of them, the boundaries with secular society became ever more rigid.

The romanticization of this enclosed, arcane world in the West began with Martin Buber's retelling of the tales of Hasidic masters at the very beginning of the twentieth century, at a time when Eastern European Jews were urbanizing and entering the working class. Some Western acculturated Jews, such as Franz Kafka and his friend Jiři Langer, were suddenly exposed to such social structures when rabbinic courts, such as that of the 'Miracle Rabbi' of Grodeck, moved to Prague during the First World War.[99] Kafka was fascinated; Langer became a follower. After the Holocaust's systematic destruction of Jewish communal life and all its religious, ethical and cultural approaches, the notion of a boundary between the state and the community as a means of resistance became even stronger. Boundaries with the secular state that had become fluid in the aftermath of the First World War became the means by which such communities reestablished their sense of integrity. What form the resistance to the dissolution of the boundary between the national state and the religious community takes is exactly what Locke had objected to: it becomes the focus of the political power of the community within and beyond its membership. And there's the rub: how can such communities negotiate the ever-shifting boundaries between themselves and the state? One way is to assume that the state is illegitimate and has no power over them, as do anti-Zionist ultra-Orthodox groups in Israel. Or to organize as a political structure to compete in the marketplace of the secular state, as in Israeli national politics and in the expansion of ultra-Orthodox communities into the counties around New York City in towns such as the new Satmar town of Kiryas Joel, in Orange County, and in Rockland County the Skver Hasid village of New Square. There the new ultra-Orthodox majority now successfully competes for state resources with the 'locals'. By the beginning of October 2020 such suburban communities north of New York City were also seeing a massive spike in

COVID-19 cases, and were being shut down systematically. What was closed were the evident sources of transmission: synagogues and religious schools.[100]

Concrete Symbols

Our focus here is one arena, that of public health, which exemplifies how difficult the now seemingly fixed but in fact ever-fluid boundaries between symbolic communities can be. We can think of no better example in which this is contested. For infectious diseases have no borders, no boundaries, except those superimposed by the state. Health seems to be a neutral sphere, but, as with all such elements, has intensive symbolic value defined by and defining the community. Indeed, this has been specifically true in the ultra-Orthodox communities where the symbolic boundaries of the community are explicit. Such communities, whether in Israel, the United States or the United Kingdom, are literally bounded by a symbolic border, an *eruv* (Hebrew for 'mixture'), drawn usually with a virtually invisible wire suspended high above neighbourhoods and delineating the area where one can 'carry' forbidden items, such as a cane or a stroller, on the Sabbath and holidays. In the United States, the establishment of such symbolic boundaries has been both highly contested and defended with the expansion of ultra-Orthodox communities beyond traditional urban areas.[101]

The *eruv* caused some communities in the New York exurbs with new and large ultra-Orthodox communities, including those with a large Jewish but not Haredi population, to see this as presenting a conflict between their secular identity and a state-sanctioned religious boundary. Similar conflicts have occurred with extensive legal battles in suburban communities in Britain such as in Barnet in northwest London.[102] That this was not part of secular Jews' symbolic register was clear, but it also seemed in conflict with their notion of being Jewish in contemporary society. One can contrast this with the rejection of masking during the pandemic in many of the ultra-Orthodox communities. The mask, however, came to stand for the imposition of civil authority on their community, even though the mask per se had only political significance in the world of Donald Trump. Trump had politicized the mask when the primary sites of infection were Democratic-controlled urban areas and the opposition to masking quickly became part of the symbolic register of the right. In Borough Park, one of the overwhelmingly ultra-Orthodox areas of New York City, 80 per cent of voters voted for Trump in 2020. In Hong Kong during the SARS pandemic in 2003, masks took a prominent place in the local symbolic register analogous to the *eruv* in Orthodox neighbourhoods, defining the boundaries of these imagined communities who visually defined themselves in support of active interventions to halt the spread of the virus.

Given that we are focusing on politically organized communities in regards to public health questions, one previous case in New York City can provide a parallel to that of COVID-19. In the early 2010s a debate arose within public health authorities in New York City, where ritual *metzitzah* among ultra-Orthodox Jews has been blamed for infant deaths from herpes. *Metzitzah b'peh*, or oral suction, drawing the blood from the circumcision wound through sucking by the ritual circumciser, had been a divisive problem among the earliest Jewish reformers. This debate about the special relationship between Jews, forms of ritual circumcision and the public's health was reflected in the *Verein der Reformfreunde* (Society for the Friends of Reform) in

Frankfurt in 1843, which said that ritual infant male circumcision was neither a religious obligation nor a symbolic act.[103] This was in response to the 8 February 1843 finding of the Frankfurt Public Health authority that circumcision had to be carried out under medical supervision. With the expanding role of medicine came further opposition; certain ritual aspects of Jewish circumcision, such as *metzitzah*, were deemed unhygienic.[104] Outbreaks of syphilis and tuberculosis from 1805 to 1865 were blamed on the ritual circumcisers. Many reformers thus advocated modifying *metzitzah* using a sponge or a glass pipette, a form in the twenty-first century advocated by Orthodox communities such as the London-based Conference of European Rabbis and the Central Council of Jews in Germany for reasons of public health. But the end result of concerns over hygiene and infection was that ritual circumcision was less and less often undertaken by acculturated Jews in Central and Western Europe from the mid-nineteenth century on.

After an outbreak that infected a number of infants with herpes, leading to seventeen cases of infant herpes and brain damage and two deaths after 2000, the New York City Board of Health passed a regulation on 12 September 2012 to require parental notification of risk, a demand that had been vociferously opposed by religious authorities who noted that the procedure has never been the cause of any possible danger to the health of the infant. According to the Board of Health, about 3,600 male infants are circumcised with direct oral suction each year and their risk of contracting herpes is estimated at roughly 1 in 4,000. The Centers for Disease Control and Prevention called the procedure unsafe and recommend against it. Indeed, some members of the Board of Health said they believed that requiring consent did not go far enough. 'It's crazy that we allow this to go on,' said Dr Joel Forman, a professor of paediatrics at Mount Sinai School of Medicine. Again, the debates centred on ritual as communitarian practice versus the health of the infant: 'This process [demanded by the Board of Health] is being created without a shred of evidence,' said Rabbi William Handler, one of a few ultra-Orthodox Jews who gathered outside the meeting in protest. 'The city is lying, and slandering compassionate rabbis.'[105] 'They feel that if their child doesn't have the *metzitzah*, he is not Jewish, so this, to them, is the most important act that they can do for their son in life,' said Dr Kenneth I. Glassberg, the director of the division of paediatric urology at Morgan Stanley Children's Hospital at New York-Presbyterian. 'Medically, I don't approve of it,' he added of the oral contact, 'but if you're asking me, "Does it cause harm?" I haven't seen enough proof that it causes harm.'[106] This is the problem with the porous boundary between theology and science: neither side can muster sufficient evidence to persuade the other, as their very concepts of evidence (understood as having symbolic value) are radically different. This was clear in present-day Israel when Moshe Morsiano, chair of the Division of Circumcision for the Chief Rabbinate of Israel, stated in his letter dated 22 April 2014 that there was no justification for avoiding *metzitzah b'peh* 'unless the mohel [ritual circumciser] has a sore in his mouth, or some infectious disease'.[107] And that, of course, based on self-reporting.

Here one needs to add the political dimension that is shaped by and shapes the symbolic register. When Bill de Blasio ran for mayor for the first time in 2013 as a Democratic candidate, his positions were generally considered to be liberal, reflecting his time on the city council. He 'viewed Ultra-Orthodox New Yorkers as a key political constituency'.[108] Needing broader support across ideological lines, he found it in 2013 in the form of the ultra-Orthodox community, to which he committed resources, for example, for childcare, which had been stripped from them by the sitting Republican mayor, Michael Bloomberg. The choice to deal with what had become both a medical and a communal question concerning the herpes infection became quickly coloured by realpolitik in New York City. De Blasio packed the city health department with allies and shifted the reporting mechanism. 'His aides spent months attempting to reach a compromise, one which when finally instituted, basically abandoned any direct outlawing of the practice and stressed only a reporting mechanism, that was honored in the breach.'[109] Only *after* a child was infected would the herpes virus be tested for its DNA and if the mohel, ritual circumciser, was found to be infected, he would be struck off the rolls. This demanded, of course, that the Board of Health report such findings (even if after the fact) and they then refused to do so, nullifying the public health demands.[110] Needless to say, numerous children were infected following this ruling. Circumcision as politics mediated the clear public health concern about infection.

When in 2014 de Blasio saw the problem in terms of an enclosed community with a local public health problem that probably could not spread beyond that community, he was at ease with suppressing information about its spread. We need to note here an obvious fact: that while any given action may spread a disease, the spread of a disease is never limited to that single practice. Oral herpes can and does transcend the boundaries of the ultra-Orthodox community in many and complex ways, as did conterminous outbreaks of measles in religious schools in 2019, which were laid at the feet of an anti-vaccination movement that certainly transcended this community. When COVID-19 appeared, the very notion of the boundary vanished. Indeed, one needs to state that the symbolic boundary of such communities, the *eruv*, which allows certain activities otherwise outlawed on the Sabbath and holidays, was valid only when such banned activities (the so-called 39 *melachot* or forms of work) were not necessary for the preservation of human life (*pikuach nefesh*). The politics of containment overrode the symbolic politics of community, at least from the point of view of the public health authorities, whose blinkered approach to the herpes epidemic suddenly vanished in the light of COVID-19 transmission. The community defended itself, aware of the earlier case, seeing the violation of the boundary between the self-policing of the community and the ability to set public health standards for the community as state-sanctioned antisemitism. De Blasio and his public health figures, who had been champions of the community in 2015, were suddenly 'Nazis'.

In Israel the party politics were even simpler. After three inconclusive elections, the shaky coalition government of Benjamin Netanyahu in 2020 had to rely on the participation of the ultra-Orthodox Shas and United Torah Judaism parties as the key to the arrangement with his opponent Benny Gantz, who became minister for defence as well as 'alternate prime minister'. One can note here that this cross-party support was undermined regularly by the necessity of controlling the pandemic, especially after Gantz was quarantined in late July 2020. It was central, for example, in forcing the public health authorities, led by the COVID czar Ronni Gamzu, to walk back their strong recommendations for greater controls in Haredi and Israeli Arab neighbourhoods to control community spread, well prior to the second national lockdown in September 2020.[111] This followed his initial failed attempt to limit the movement of yeshiva students from entering the country, especially from lands with a very high positivity rate, a rate which in August was relatively under control in Israel.[112] By the end of December 2020 the government was in disarray, the pandemic was radically spiking and a new election, the fourth in two years, was called for March 2021. The inability to control the spread of the virus in the Haredi community exacerbated a national public health crisis as cases increased and vaccine resistance was more pronounced there; indeed, as many as three-quarters of those in the community stated they would not take the vaccine. The public health measures continued to be seen from within the ultra-Orthodox community as an attack by 'Nazis'.[113]

So, we have the instrumentalization of a specific moment in history, the Holocaust, through which the ultra-Orthodox communities now define themselves as victims in their opposition to the public health actions of a Jewish state, labelled as the 'Nazis'. Other anti-masking, anti-lockdown political groups, including in Germany, identify themselves with the victims of the Holocaust because of their political position. For these different groups, the Holocaust is a vector for pushing their otherwise different political agendas. (This is analogous to how British Imperialism and the Opium War have served as a vector for the emergence of Chinese nationalism ever since the turn of the twentieth century. They are evoked over and again by the Chinese state as well as different social groups in times of radically differing political crisis, such as during the current pandemic, as we discussed in Chapter Two.) This occurs simultaneously with attacks on Jews by the ultra-right that are also opposed to the same public health actions. This takes place in a wide-range of nation-states, from Poland to Hungary to the United States, with the ultra-right employing the vocabulary of classic antisemitism to describe their own victimization. The

August 2017 attacks in Charlottesville, Virginia, on the financier George Soros as the Rothschild of today manipulating the world to establish Jewish hegemony, and the Neo-Nazis' shouts that the 'Jews will not replace us' with racial inferiors, frame the debates about COVID-19 and placing the blame. It is not incidental that well-poisoning becomes the go-to image of radically false accusations of blame, including against ultra-Orthodox communities. The difficulty we have is that exactly those communities, having struggled with their political boundaries, use this very atmosphere as the protective camouflage to defend the community's autonomy. Placing the blame is thus a double-edged sword. It provides for some in the nation-state a well-worn and comfortable enemy, already clearly defined as pernicious and vile, and, for those communities so identified, a means to defend their own boundaries against state encroachment – even, or especially, where encroachment is so vital, such as in the area of the public's health, where no boundaries can exist among symbolically defined communities. The virus is symbol-blind but it is also boundary-neutral, no matter how fervently such boundaries are imagined to exist.

4

ANXIETY IN THE AFRICAN AMERICAN
AND BAME COMMUNITIES

One of the striking patterns in examining the African American community (and as we shall see, in complex ways, also the BAME communities in Britain) and COVID-19 is the set of assumptions about attitudes towards infection, vaccination and risk. Too often they are read as artefacts of the historical treatment of these communities. This is layered upon the quotidian experienced reality of communities of colour today as being at the greatest risk for COVID-19 and even in terms of treatment, as Professor Lisa Cooper of the Johns Hopkins University noted, 'the unprecedented stress on the healthcare system during the coronavirus crisis could exacerbate existing biases among already overloaded hospital staff.'[1] A recent detailed examination by the Pew Foundation revealed that 'Black Americans are especially likely to say they know someone who has been hospitalized or died as a result of having the coronavirus: 71 percent say this, compared with smaller shares of Hispanic (61 percent), White (49 percent) and Asian-American (48 percent) adults.'[2] We need to understand the double bind that individuals who identify with this community found themselves in, at least according to many commentators, during the pandemic. They were the most at risk but also the most fearful of allopathic interventions. They were the most likely to become ill but also the most likely to transmit the virus to others. Little mention is made of the ancillary causes of anxiety evident in the disparities highlighted by the pandemic: loss of employment and housing, inability to afford access to healthcare because of diminished employment or poverty, employment in low-paid but 'essential' services, multigenerational households, living in areas of increased air and water pollution, and so on.[3] As is clear from the public record, the health of such communities in 2020 is dire: 'Black and Native American women are more likely to die in childbirth than other groups. Blacks and Hispanics who are in pain are less likely to receive treatment than White patients.' George McKinney, senior pastor of Impact Global Ministries in Valencia Park, California, goes on to observe: 'They're not taking care of us in terms of our health care. We're not taken seriously when we have pain and discomfort, and that's documented. So those things add up to a distrust of the medical community and the government.'[4] And to quote from the Pew Report again, the corollary is rejecting allopathic medicine: 'Black Americans continue to stand out as less inclined to get vaccinated than other racial and ethnic groups: 42 percent would do so, compared with 63 percent of Hispanic and 61 percent of white adults.' It is no accident that when the first vaccines (Pfizer-BioNTech) were made available in the United States on 14 December 2020, the exemplary individuals shown getting vaccinated in the media were African American. The first was Sandra Lindsay, 'the director of critical care nursing at the Long Island Jewish Medical Center, [who] said she wanted to lead by example – particularly as a Black woman who understands the legacy of unequal and racist medical treatment and experimentation on people of color'. She stated it was not vital 'to be the first one to take the vaccine, but to inspire people who look like me, who are skeptical in general about taking vaccines'.[5] And yet Lindsay is hardly the stereotyped economically and socially marginalized African American that dominates the reporting on COVID-19. Black women have entered the middle class as professionals in greater numbers in the past decades than Black men.[6]

We wish to raise a counter-reading of the cause of this anxiety. It has been claimed that it is inherently different from that articulated by the more traditional anti-vaxxers. These communities of anti-vaxxers, it is claimed, have had their middle-class sensibilities driven by the ubiquity of 'bad science' on social media as well as the simple historical fact that their generation of suburban dwellers was never exposed to the mortality and morbidity of childhood infectious diseases from measles to polio.[7] Thus the claim is that communities of colour have a 'valid' anxiety about allopathic medicine, while suburban middle-class 'soccer moms and dads' do not. Charles Blow in the *New York Times* summarized this as a statement of fact: 'The unfortunate American fact is that Black people in this country have been well-trained, over centuries, to distrust both the government and the medical establishment on the issue of health care.'[8] Let us clearly state that the range of historic medical mistreatments of minorities in the United States and the United Kingdom is clear, but we would argue that it is not a 'community memory' of such mistreatments but their constant evocation in the context of COVID-19 that creates a symbolic register defining the risk confronting these communities and simultaneously generating anxiety within them. What is vital is to understand that such cases, real as they are, were excavated and are reproduced regularly to generate a pseudo-collective memory, one which is instrumentalized by post-colonial public historians, the media, popular culture and social networks to create an image of the danger to the African American Black community, in the case of the United States, and the BAME community, in the United Kingdom, from *all* medical research and practice.

We can interpolate here for a moment into our overall argument an observation concerning placing the blame in this context. It is clear that African Americans and BAME communities, while suffering the greatest morbidity and mortality in 2020, have not themselves been the target of blame. This is supported by Nexis searches for 'Black/African American', 'BAME', 'COVID' and 'blame/cause' from 1 March 2020 to 1 March 2021. It is uncertain whether this is because the pandemic overlapped with the worldwide Black Lives Matter protests in the wake of deaths of numerous African Americans over the course of 2020 or whether the overwhelming catastrophes that have befallen communities of colour in the United States make such attacks uncomfortable or at least unprofitable for racists to exploit. Yet at the back of everyone's mind is the mass hysteria in the United States associated with the eleven cases of Ebola that were registered in the country during 2014 and the constant screed against Haitians during the 1980s and '90s accusing them of having brought HIV/AIDS into the United States in 1982, part of the quartet of those blamed for the spread of the virus, the '4-Hs': Homosexuals, Heroin addicts, Haemophiliacs and Haitians.[9] In the case of Ebola, those impacted were almost exclusively found among White medical specialists, having been exposed serving in public health roles in the Republic of the Congo. The fear that was aimed at them was as potentially the 'source' of a wider American outbreak of this so-labelled 'African plague'. It was 'Africa', not African Americans, that triggered the fear. As for the anti-Haitian sentiment decades earlier in regards to HIV/AIDS, Haiti became the scene for the demonization of 'Patient Zero', Gaëtan Dugas, in Randy Shilt's *And the Band Played On: Politics, People, and the AIDS Epidemic* in 1987.[10] Texts do matter especially in this regard: Shilt's best-selling account made 'Haiti' again a byword for risk in the twenty-first century.

One can note an alternative case in the United Kingdom. There, as elsewhere, 'race', 'ethnicity' and 'religion' turn out to be easily conflated, just as in the United States, 'class' and 'race' seem to be interchangeable. Muslims have been blamed for *purposely* transmitting COVID-19 in India, as we have discussed in Chapter One, and this false narrative seems to have touched a nerve in the UK. In August 2020 limited lockdowns were announced in areas such as Darwen, Bradford and Leicester, which have significant Islamic populations. As Rabnawaz Akbar, a Labour Party councillor in Manchester, observed,

> The timing . . . focused people's minds [on Muslims]. [The government] have done it on the eve of Eid [leading people to think] it must be the Muslim community's fault . . . You see how people would have come to the assumption. [The government] have done it without thinking but of course, they're highlighting a particular demographic. And people are angry and now that anger is focused on a particular community.[11]

These remonstrations echo much of the rhetoric in the ultra-Orthodox Jewish community concerning lockdowns and blame. Yet the argument on the part of the public health authorities in the UK, like those in New York City, is that this is simply where in late August 2020 the increases had been greatest, even though individual members of parliament blamed the BAME communities for disregarding the guidelines because of their religious practices. The focus in the United States, however, has been on African Americans and their potential anxiety about COVID-19 testing and vaccination.

Thus, if we search Nexis for 'COVID-19', 'African American' and 'vaccination', we find that after 1 March 2020 there were in excess of 10,000 citations, the maximum number reported by the database. There is a red thread in these accounts which is noteworthy. In March 2020, as a potential trial for vaccines was imagined, but thought of as in the distant future, this historicizing theme was clear. Kawsar R. Talaat, an assistant professor in International Health at the Johns Hopkins University, commented that diversity would be essential for any human trials of a potential vaccine. By diversity, Talaat meant the inclusion of African Americans, not only because of the need for genetic and developmental diversity (which would include a wide range of subjects from women to children as well as other genetic haplotypes) but because of the specific history of the treatment of African Americans by allopathic medicine. 'We've come a long, long way from the earliest days of vaccine trials, the earliest being James Phipps being given cowpox to protect him against smallpox without his consent.' The central case however is not Edward Jenner and the cowpox vaccine but the infamous mid-twentieth-century Tuskegee Study of syphilis among a group of African American men, which we shall discuss in much greater detail below: 'The FDA acknowledged, however, that some people may hesitate to participate in research because of "historical mistreatment" of human subjects as in the Tuskegee Study, which began in 1932 and continued for 40 years.'[12]

By the beginning of December 2020, after the announcement of two successful vaccines for COVID-19, Anna Durbin, principal investigator at the Johns Hopkins Center for Immunization Research, stressed that to determine a vaccine candidate's efficacy it must be tested 'in different populations because they want to make sure it works in the groups most affected by COVID-19 . . .

In Baltimore, that means signing up some 300 Black residents for the AstraZeneca trial alone.' Her colleague Kawsar R. Talaat again resumed her anxiety about the historical experiences of Blacks in regard to the history of testing and of treatment:

> Historically, medical research has not treated these popu-lations well . . . The Tuskegee [syphilis study] comes up in pretty much in every conversation that we have. It is still very fresh on the minds of people, and it's something that we have to address – the huge mistakes and huge abuses.[13]

'Fresh on the minds of people', but from what source? Certainly from the mass and social media during the pandemic, not from some collective 'folk memory'.

Indeed, at virtually the very same moment, on 2 December 2020, the former president Barack Obama gave a pre-taped interview with SiriusXM host Joe Madison to promote his new memoir, *A Promised Land*. When asked about African Americans potentially being sceptical about taking a COVID-19 vaccine given past medical experiments on the community, President Obama said he would 'absolutely' take the vaccine himself:

> And I understand, historically, everything dating back all the way to the Tuskegee experiments and so forth, why the African-American community would have some skepti-cism. But the fact of the matter is, is that vaccines are why we don't have polio anymore. And they're the reason why we don't have a whole bunch of kids dying from measles, and smallpox, and diseases that used to decimate an entire populations and communities . . . And I promise you that when it's been made for people who are less at risk, I

will be taking it. I may end up taking it on TV or having it filmed, just so that people know that I trust this science, and what I don't trust is getting COVID. I think at this point, particularly in the African-American community, we are – African Americans, Hispanics, Native Americans – we have the highest death rates from this thing, and are most exposed and most vulnerable, in part because we have a lot of preexisting conditions.[14]

Yes, the African American community has been extraordinarily impacted by COVID-19, as these commentators also have noted, but we would argue that it also was the subject of a direct campaign of focused historical information that has heightened anxieties by evoking the worst-case scenarios from the past. The reality is that communities of colour were and are disproportionately impacted by COVID-19 and that health disparities between these communities and the White majority do exist, as do higher rates of preexisting conditions. Yet the evocation of these historical cases has the effect of relativizing today's actual social cause and marginalizing the cause of such anxiety, which is rooted in the ongoing, systemic racism of today's Western societies, by stressing the historical victimization of these communities in medical research and treatment. These too have a history, but the examples become untethered to any specific historical events, rather being exemplary of the systemic racism with which American medical practice, theory and delivery is clearly intertwined.[15] The difficulty is that in doing this one is exemplifying the wrong aspects to be feared: experiment or exploitation, rather than access and equal treatment. The analogy, as we have seen, is the use of the Holocaust as the model within which the ultra-Orthodox Jewish community understands its treatment by state authorities during the COVID-19 pandemic in the USA, the UK and Israel. Antisemitism and racism are as real in the present as they were in the past, but faulty analogies to specific cases such as these are intended to generate fear.

A Distorted Mirror

When being African American comes to be identified with being ill or at risk, fear morphs into placing blame. But it is also the case that the evocation of vulnerability within such stereotyped communities plays a major role. The case, as we noted, that is most often cited concerning Black communities is that of the so-called Tuskegee Experiment. Nexis registers almost 1,500 references to this and COVID-19 after 1 March 2020. One summarized the situation as, 'In perhaps the most egregious example, U.S. public health officials in the 1930s began a study in which syphilis was left untreated in Black men. Known colloquially as the Tuskegee Experiment, the study didn't end until 1972, and has become shorthand among African Americans for a legacy of racism and mistreatment in the medical industry.'[16] In point of fact the study had its roots in a generalized claim that minorities responded to various forms of infectious disease in a way that was radically different from (read: inferior to) Whites.[17] This led to the long-standing claims that 'ritually observant' Jews had greater immunity from tuberculosis and that 'promiscuous' Blacks suffered from syphilis to a much lesser degree than Whites. Neither, by the way, is true. The study was initially supported by the Rosenwald Fund, founded by Julius Rosenwald, the Jewish president of Sears, Roebuck & Co., in 1912.[18] It was one of the major supporters of both African American education and health. Its intent was to examine syphilis seroprevalence in the American South and it was 'characterized as a humanitarian effort to benefit the health of rural African Americans. The study reported extraordinarily high rates of positive Wassermann tests, even among children.'[19] While the initial intent may have been to examine the 'normal' course of the disease, it is clear that its impact was to stress that the poor health of Blacks in the South was a risk to this source of cheap labour. The 'white man's burden' of colonialism, with the concomitant rise of tropical medicine, was clearly paralleled by such undertakings in the Jim Crow South. Yet such views on Black health disparities, no matter what their source, were also very much in line with those of Booker T. Washington, the founder of the Tuskegee Institute, also underwritten by Rosenwald, who launched National Negro Health Week with a lecture in 1914. 'Without health, and until we reduce the high death rate, it will be impossible for us to have permanent success in business, in property getting, in acquiring education, or to show other evidences of progress.'[20] The following year, the year of his death, the U.S. Public Health Service officially adopted the week as a national public health event. Thus the Tuskegee Institute remained the natural home of such a study of normal African American responses to disease. Paul Goldberger's more or less contemporaneous public health studies of pellagra were also similar attempts to counter such racial specificity, looking at poor Whites and poor Blacks in the South and the impact of poverty, rather than supposed bad character, on the aetiology of the disease.[21] It is at this moment, the age of the Muckrakers, of reformers such as Ida B. Wells and Jacob Riis, that social medicine became fashionable, hence the emphasis on the link between poverty and poor health.[22]

The Rosenwald Fund abandoned the study in 1932 as the state of Alabama refused to match its funds. In that year, as the

CDC notes, the 'Public Health Service, working with the Tuskegee Institute, began a study to record the natural history of syphilis in hopes of justifying treatment programs for blacks. It came to be called the "Tuskegee Study of Untreated Syphilis in the Negro Male."'[23] The Public Health Service that continued the study was a paramilitary organization within the U.S. Surgeon General's office and its initial task was to guard the American borders against diseased foreign elements infiltrating from abroad, including across the Mexican border.[24] It also functioned in the new American colonies from Cuba to the Philippines, captured from Spain in the 1890s.[25] That it had its own agenda in continuing the study is without doubt. It was certainly no longer interested in looking at the 'normality' of infectious processes in African Americans, but rather at the pathological difference and the sexualized danger imputed to the Black body.[26]

It is important to note both the claims of the initial study and the date. The claims were that Blacks and Whites suffered equally from the disease, but that Blacks were somehow less impacted by it, a claim made about a wide range of minorities at the time. Treatment options for syphilis in 1932 were limited and often unsuccessful. Salvarsan (arsphenamine) was far from being a 'magic bullet', which it was hailed as at the time. It had been developed by the German researcher Paul Ehrlich in 1909. Not only was the drug expensive but the treatment course was long, over two years, and could cause fateful side effects, even death. It was only long after the Second World War, with the general availability of antibiotics such as penicillin, that the treatment of venereal diseases became commonplace. By then the Rosenwald Foundation had long abandoned the study, which was assumed by the U.S. Public Health Service. They then purposefully allowed the now treatable disease to go untreated both in the subjects and their families, including a number of children born with congenital syphilis.

This horrific fact was first made public by Peter Buxtun, a Czech Jewish refugee whistleblower in the U.S. Public Health Service, in 1972. He leaked the details of the study directly to the media after the Public Health Service refused for years to act on his complaints. The scandal resulted in a Senate investigation, which in turn led to major improvements in informed consent with the issuance of the government's Belmont Report (1976). The discussion about informed consent had been only introduced in the United States after the Second World War.[27] But informed consent had been a hot-button issue in Imperial Germany, with clear analogies to the Tuskegee Experiment. In 1898 there was public outrage concerning the research of Albert Neisser, who had discovered the pathogen responsible for gonorrhoea, when it was revealed that he had involuntarily infected his female subjects, who were prostitutes, with syphilis during his experiments with a treatment for the disease.[28] However, globally it was only after the Nuremberg Doctors Trial of 1946–7 that a universal standard for medical experimentation began to evolve. The horrors of the Nazi concentration camps demanded a rethinking of human experimentation. It was only with the public exposure of what came to be called the Jewish Chronic Disease Hospital Case in 1963 that the idea of informed consent was fixed within American public awareness.[29] And that only because of the massive coverage in the media, from the *New York Times* to local newspapers, of the injection of live cancer cells into Jewish Holocaust survivors and others, who were thus used as guinea pigs for research into their immunological response.[30] The Jewish Chronic Disease Hospital Case, however, had virtually no impact on the careers of the researchers involved, even with the powerful evocation of Nazi medical experiments on Jews during this public discussion. Yet as a result of the publicity in the 1970s the Tuskegee Experiment was immediately closed down.[31] The difference, of course, was the post-war integration of Jews into American society, with the social capital of the Holocaust in the background, pace Peter Novick, and the concomitant rise of the civil rights movement during the same period.[32] But its public impact came later when in 1981 James H. Jones published his best-selling study of the Tuskegee experiments, which in turn led to David Feldshuh's Pulitzer Prize-nominated play, *Miss Evers' Boys*, in 1992 and then to a seven-issue Marvel comic book series in 2003, *Truth: Red, White, and Black*.[33] It became a core element in the symbolic register of the Black community in regard to all forms of allopathic medicine.

We have selected the Tuskegee Experiment and its reception as our initial focus in the construction of a symbolic register of health and disease, but there are many more examples that are cited in the recent discussions of Blacks and COVID-19 vaccination, such as J. Marion Sims's abuse of female slaves in his mid-nineteenth-century gynaecological research, which led to the removal of his statue from Central Park in New York City in 2018.[34] In the twenty-first century the case of Henrietta Lacks, whose 'immortal' cell line was taken by Johns Hopkins researchers in 1951 and used without her consent for scientific research, became a mass cultural phenomenon. The so-called 'HeLa' cells remain today a vital research tool for cancer researchers and have aided researchers in developing vaccines against polio and human papillomavirus. This case was the subject of Rebecca Skloot's best-selling book of 2010, which remained for months on the *New York Times* best-seller list, as well as a 2017 made-for-TV film starring and executive produced by Oprah Winfrey.[35]

All became part of a web of symbols, for even though their historical reach is from the antebellum South to the 1930s to the 1950s, they are used to comment on the state of access to allopathic medicine today, as we can see in a statement by Professor Lisa Cooper of the Johns Hopkins University: 'Racial discrimination in the world of medicine has a particularly gruesome history in America, stretching back to the gynecological experiments of J. Marion Sims on enslaved women in the 1840s, to the infamous Tuskegee Experiment and the case of Henrietta Lacks.'[36] But the reality is quite different, as Reed Tuckson, a doctor and a former Washington, DC, health director, observed: 'We are taking great pains to help folks understand that what existed in the 1930s is very different today, in 2020. That there are research scientists of color who are in positions of authority all across the research and medical enterprise.'[37] To this one can add the fact that since 1993 the CDC and the FDA have mandated the inclusion of people of colour and women as test subjects in all such studies. In the UK the MHRA (Medicines and Healthcare Products Regulatory Agency) does likewise. While access to treatment may be limited in the United States by economic and geographical factors (and in the UK by the so-called 'postcode lottery' of the NHS), research studies must now include these marginalized communities.

Instrumentalizing History

Is it the history or its reception that is driving this anxiety? Do historical texts (and the echoes in social media) provide a reality that may well have its roots in the past but are read as acting in the future? We can think of benign examples as well as those that poison the public well. George W. Bush sitting at his ranch in Texas reading an advance copy of John M. Barry's *The Great*

Influenza in 2005, which motivates him to develop a comprehensive pandemic plan that, as is often stated, helped structure federal responses to future outbreaks.[38] Yet the reality in 2005 was actually quite different, as in John M. Barry's account at the time:

> Barry, author of 'The Great Influenza,' said that he too had been a Bush critic. But his views have not deterred the administration from seeking his advice on the potential for another pandemic like the 1918 outbreak that claimed millions of lives worldwide. Although Barry was not aware that the president planned to read the book, he said he had been consulting off and on with senior administration officials since its release in February 2004 . . . A central theme of Barry's book is that the 1918 outbreak was exacerbated in America by the government's attempts to minimize its significance, partly to avoid undermining efforts to prevail in World War i. 'One lesson is to absolutely take it seriously,' Barry said. 'I'm not a great fan of the Bush administration, but I think they are doing that.'

What is vital is that this account becomes part of the textual framing of the COVID-19 narratives.[39] If only Donald J. Trump had read a book, things would have been different! Does history, or at least consuming those texts analysing and documenting history ('Ceci n'est pas une pipe'), really play a role in constituting a community response and how does this impact on both compliance and self-image in these communities? Here one would normally misquote George Santayana bemoaning in his *The Life of Reason* how 'savages . . . [whose] infancy is perpetual' cannot retain any sense of 'the past [and] are condemned to repeat it', echoing Hegel on the Africans, rather than Karl Marx contrasting

Napoleon Bonaparte with his pathetic nephew Napoleon III, for many of these cases were first tragedies and their citation now has become a dangerous farce.[40] This seems to be a commonplace in prejudging how a community would respond (or indeed has responded).

But what happens when the proliferation of the accounts of victimization in the African American community seems to argue that one should rely on past events rather than present realities? Let us begin by arguing that there are many Black communities in the United States (and in Britain), each of which may have different yet seemingly overlapping symbolic registers concerning health and disease. The difference between Lisa Cooper and Reed Tuckson is the difference between seeing the historical record as shaping the present and the present being a contrast with the past. One of the best studies of the framing of Rebecca Skloot's book on Henrietta Lacks noted that it made accessible to the 'general public what were once arcane bioethical debates regarding the relationships between public science, patient autonomy, and the politics of race, class, and gender'.[41] One can state the same of James H. Jones's book on the Tuskegee Experiment or Deirdre Cooper Owens's study of Sims. But the reader's reception is also vital. When we look at elite texts (and their mass cultural spin-offs) we see a history of medical malfeasance superimposed on the African American community by a dominant White society. What we do not see are the academics exploring Black victimhood to frame the past in contrast with the present, for good or for ill. The social reality of COVID-19 is that it has revealed the health disparities in the United States along economic fault lines. And it is clear that race and ethnicity are often indicators that follow those same lines or indeed create them. But the symbolic register of such distinctions is that Black Americans are at risk not only from the virus but from the medical interventions that could mitigate it. This is a very different argument from the one that states that poor people (and today even lower middle-class people) who cannot afford medical care, who live in communities (urban or rural) where healthcare is simply not available, are at much greater risk, not from the actions of the healthcare system, but from its absence. This fear of abandonment is laid by many today at the feet of a historical disparity of treatment and callous disregard for Black health in the cases spanning the nineteenth to the mid-twentieth centuries. Here the repetition of such cases as evidence for the contemporary and existential flaws in the American healthcare system masks its true problems.

Vaccination of minority populations in the United States is a priority of the Joseph Biden administration, which also acknowledges the extraordinary cost of vaccinating everyone in the United States and its dependencies. But this is not a level playing field. Here we can mention some glaring disparities in the very limited publicly funded federal healthcare available in 2021 for the poor and the marginal: the limited expansion of Medicaid (health access for the poor), as well as the chronic underfunding of the Indian Health Service, all impact the access of people of colour. A quarter of all veterans in the poorly managed Veterans Administration's public healthcare system are minorities, a proportion that will increase to almost 40 per cent in the next decades.

And that list can easily be expanded down to the local level. These endemic problems are certainly more central to the real experiences of African Americans in 2020 than the history of Black victimization by allopathic medical research. By focusing on the latter, one exacerbates the fear and the anxiety that is real but deflects from the existing and pernicious problems of the implementation of healthcare across these communities.

African American Voices on the Right

One needs to add that by late December 2020, those African Americans supporting the outgoing President Trump in the media signed on to a rather different response to the desirability of interventions for COVID-19. Trump had met with these Black supporters in the White House on 26 February 2020 as the pandemic had taken hold. He spent the meeting complaining about his press coverage, stating that the risk from COVID-19 was 'low' and listening to his Black supporters advocate his strong leadership. One of them, Candace Owens, then published, in September 2020, a strongly pro-Trump book prior to the election, *Blackout: How Black America Can Make Its Second Escape from the Democratic Plantation*.[42] In it she castigated, following Trump, most of the interventions concerning social controls for the pandemic. On the approval of the initial vaccines, she tweeted on 9 December 2020 that 'the same people that are out here yelling "my body my choice" will be telling you that the government has a right to force vaccinate you for a virus that has a 99% survival rate.'[43] Putting aside for a moment the equation of being pro-choice (pro-abortion) with vaccination, the irony is, of course that the central problem of the pandemic is its infectious nature, not the question of individual autonomy or choice. Owens, insisting that she would not take any vaccination, tweeted: 'It's pretty incredible to consider that right now governments are like "in order to keep you safe, we need to impoverish you, imprison you, force mask and vaccinate you, plus separate you from your family." And there are millions of people out there that are just like "okay!"' Owens had already on 15 December 2020 condemned both Dr Anthony Fauci and Bill Gates, both of whom had been advocating mass vaccination, as 'pure evil' and tools of the pharmaceutical industry.[44]

Such sentiments had been already merged with the claim of a global medical conspiracy by two of Trump's other African American media advocates also present at his 26 February meeting, Diamond (Ineitha Lynnette Hardaway) and Silk (Herneitha Rochelle Hardaway Richardson), who in April damned Gates. 'Kudos if you make your vaccines for people and you want to help people, but I have a problem receiving any vaccine from any entity, especially anybody like Bill Gates who pushed for population control. The same thing that Margaret Sanger pushed for.'[45] By 12 December 2020 they were echoing the conservative line about individual autonomy espoused by Fox News commentators such as Tucker Carlson.[46] What is absent in this rather unremarkable evocation of conspiracy from the right wing is any reference to the specificity of medical crimes against African Americans, because that would stress the very different circumstances Blacks were in during and prior to the pandemic. Such a reference would be a tangible sign of systemic racism in American society, which is why it has been appropriated, for good or for ill, to focus the attention on the anxieties of African Americans concerning vaccination.

To this we can add a claim by an African American physician and pastor, Stella Immanuel, who was educated in Cameroon and licenced in Texas. She led a demonstration by a group called 'America's Frontline Doctors' in front of the u.s. Supreme Court in July 2020 in which she supported the use of the anti-malaria drug hydroxychloroquine, which Trump had pushed as a miracle cure for the coronavirus. During the press conference she stated, 'Nobody needs to get sick. This virus has a cure – it is called hydroxychloroquine. I have treated over 350 patients and not had one death.' Opposing face masks, she was the perfect spokesperson for Trump's views, and he acknowledged that she was 'very impressive' as she had had 'tremendous success with hundreds of different patients, I thought her voice was an important voice but I know nothing about her'.[47] He shared a video of her statement. At the same moment he had forced the u.s. Food and Drug Administration (FDA) to issue an emergency use authorization (EUA) for the drug on 27 April. The federal government purchased millions of doses of this unproven – and, as it later turned out, extremely dangerous – drug to be employed in Veterans Administration hospitals. The EUA was revoked on 15 June after serious side effects were documented. Once the mRNA vaccines were announced, Immanuel fell back into the Christian anti-vaxxers' rhetoric. She stated in a video that they '"are evil and are used to make blacks sterile in order to depopulate them" . . . For her the pandemic is a lie and "the processes of taking the vaccines . . . the mark of the beast"'.[48]

It is clear that African Americans do not speak with a single voice, and neither do they fear the same things. At that moment Immanuel was no longer the spokesperson for the anti-science group. Dr Simone Gold, a White, Jewish emergency-room physician who was part of the insurrection at the Capitol on 6 January 2021, had taken on that role.[49] Immanuel's religious rhetoric, speaking about 'demon sperm', quickly came to be widely satirized on the web. At a demonstration in front of the CDC in Atlanta on 13 December 2020, Gold advocated a more libertarian view, stating that such health measures were state 'coercion': 'We will fight against any experimental therapy being forced on anyone.'[50] She articulated this sentiment in a lecture to the mob in the Rotunda on 6 January 2021, surrounded by marauding rioters. She, along with another member of her group, was sub-sequently charged with 'entering a restricted building, violent entry and disorderly conduct' after her image appeared on an FBI wanted poster.

BAME

While there is a belief that the response to and in minority com-munities in the West is more or less equivalent, the symbolic register among such communities reflects local as well as global assumptions. In the UK, early in the pandemic, mounting evi-dence also began to show that Black, Asian and minority ethnic communities, under the label of BAME, were not only dying at a dis-proportionate rate but were and still are overexposed to COVID-19 and more likely to suffer the economic consequences.[51] By spring 2020 the Institute for Fiscal Studies published a study noting that 'per-capita COVID-19 hospital deaths are highest among the black Caribbean population and three times those of the white British majority. Some minority groups – including Pakistanis and black Africans – have seen similar numbers of hospital deaths per capita to the population average, while Bangladeshi fatalities are lower.' What was striking was the age differential.

> Once you take account of age and geography, most minor-ity groups 'should' have fewer deaths per capita than the white British majority. While many minority groups live disproportionately in areas such as London, Glasgow, and Birmingham, which have more COVID-19 deaths, most minorities are also younger on average than the population as a whole, which should make them less vulnerable.[52]

These communities are not only overall sicker than the majority, but all sectors, the young as well as the old, who were assumed to be most at risk, are disproportionately impacted.

Nexis lists well over the maximum 10,000 hits for 'COVID' and 'BAME' after 1 March 2020. But the focus shifted from victimization from outside communities of colour to their own resistance. As early as 4 March 2020 Kevin Courtney, joint general secretary for the National Education Union, stressed the 'very worrying victimization of BAME staff and students' already present. Weyman Bennett, joint national secretary for the organization Stand Up to Racism, saw the rise in racist attacks as indicative of a potentially fragmenting society.

> Where a disease originates does not explain the disease . . . I was on the train from Wimbledon, where people left the carriage because there was a Chinese man with a mask on it. [It is] unusual because people are saying 'I have been attacked because people say I am bringing disease' and that is kind of worrying really.[53]

This became, as it was in the United States, a political talking point. On 23 March 2020 Hina Bokhari, councillor for the London borough of Merton and Liberal Democrat London Assembly candidate, repeated many of the common assertions affirming the community spread of the disease:

> People from South Asian, African, and Caribbean backgrounds are more likely to suffer from diabetes, putting them at greater risk of suffering from harmful symptoms of Covid-19. Additionally, elderly people from South and East Asian backgrounds score worse on the 'health related

quality of life for those people of 65 and older.' Many from BAME backgrounds also face higher risks of transmitting or contracting the virus, due to living in extended families, or through regular attendance of places of worship.[54]

In Parliament in April 2020, at the request of the Labour leader Keir Starmer, Baroness Doreen Lawrence, the mother of Stephen Lawrence, a Black teenager murdered in a racist attack in 1993, led a review for the Labour Party to investigate the reasons. The review concluded that

> Covid-19 has thrived on inequalities that have long scarred British society. Black, Asian and minority ethnic people are more likely to work in frontline or shutdown sectors which have been overexposed to Covid-19, more likely to have co-morbidities which increase the risk of serious illness and more likely to face barriers to accessing healthcare. Black, Asian and minority ethnic people have also been subject to disgraceful racism as some have sought to blame different communities for the spread of the virus.

The review also showed that

> the Covid-19 pandemic has fueled racism as some have sought to blame Black, Asian and minority ethnic communities for spreading the virus . . . This also appears to be feeding into the enforcement of restrictions by public authorities. Liberty has found that police forces in England and Wales are up to seven times more likely to fine Black, Asian and minority ethnic people for violating lockdown rules.[55]

This is a crisis, according to the report, resulting from long-standing 'structural racism' that has worsened since 2010 as the Conservatives have implemented a range of policies to intentionally and openly create a 'hostile environment' in the UK. The report called for an end to structural racism as a solution to prevent such an 'avoidable crisis' happening again.[56] This was in anticipation of a statement by the Conservative government's adviser on ethnicity, Dr Raghib Ali, who argued that there was not sufficient evidence that systemic racism was the cause of the increased risk to BAME communities of COVID-19. Indeed, he noted that 'while studies often differed in their conclusions, the older people are, and where they lived, were two of the biggest factors behind the increased risks.' Yet he also argued that only a 'small part' of the increased risk for these groups was yet to be explained.[57] One needs to note that while structural racism is a reality and exists in the UK as it does in the United States, the economic reality of those BAME individuals sitting in Parliament accounts for their lesser risk than those in ghettoized racial neighbourhoods in London or Glasgow.[58] Who labels is as important as who is labelled.

Raghib Ali's views prefigured the Conservative government's Commission on Race and Ethnic Disparities report, released on 31 March 2021, which heralded the fact that 'we no longer see a Britain where the system is deliberately rigged against ethnic minorities. The impediments and disparities do exist, they are varied, and ironically very few of them are directly to do with racism.' But it is also clear that this report was a direct response to the pandemic, as it had been 'carried out under the shadow of the COVID-19 pandemic, and the evidence that some ethnic minority groups have faced a disproportionate impact from the virus'. The report claims that such accounts are merely 'overly pessimistic narratives, heightened by the COVID-19 pandemic, [which have] been on race and health. The increased age-adjusted risk of death from COVID-19 in Black and South Asian groups has widely been reported as being due to racism – and as exacerbating existing health inequalities.' But we know better, the government experts opine, as 'most of the causes of health inequalities (deprivation, tobacco, alcohol, unhealthy diet and physical inactivity) are not due to differences in healthcare' but, and here we must extrapolate, to the faults of the ill and the dead, a view similar to the one William Hogarth projected in his 1751 engraving *Gin Lane*. Had they only had better jobs, neither smoked nor imbibed, eaten organic and fresh rather than processed food, had they jogged and biked, they could have survived the virus. Yet the authors also argue that 'genetic risk factors' along with these 'cultural' and 'behavioural' factors have predetermined any differential in mortality and morbidity. No systemic racism: just cultural, social and biological inferiority. The conclusion noted, 'too many people in the progressive and anti-racism movements seem reluctant to acknowledge their own past achievements, and they offer solutions based on the binary divides of the past which often misses the point of today's world.' And these people also seem to put too much weight on the racial and economic disparities that were evident in the more than 150,000 pandemic deaths in the UK by the date the report was issued, one of the highest per capita death rates in Europe.

For the Conservative government and its appointed Commission on Race and Ethnic Disparities institutional racism does not exist in 'multicultural Britain': success in education has 'transformed British society over the last 50 years into one offering far greater opportunities for all'. This seems to echo the overall narrative underpinning the Boris Johnson government and twenty-first-century Britain as it reconfigured its global role after Brexit: it cherishes the ghost of its imperialist past by celebrating the British abolitionists who helped to end the British participation in the slave trade and deliberately avoids acknowledging that Britain was one of the most successful slave-trading countries as well as having committed gross violations of human rights in its former colonies well after the end of slavery. On the contrary, 'the Caribbean experience which speaks to the slave period [was not only] about profit and suffering but how culturally African people transformed themselves into a re-modelled African/Britain'. Slavery made good British citizens, after a while. Even if the overwhelming majority of Britons who have died in the current pandemic are ethnic minorities, since the dead cannot speak and hence have no voice, such disparities, according to the Johnson Conservative government and its Commission, could not have resulted directly from racism. In addition to geography, family influence, socio-economic background, the report argues that culture and religion had 'more significant impact on life chances than the existence of racism'. Their clarion call for the deprived struggling to survive the pandemic was to stop being haunted by historic racism, as they 'need to overcome the legacy of mistrust' that could be a barrier to success: get modern and get education, and achieve better health and economic outcomes, without any need for state intervention.

When the first vaccines were made generally available in Britain in the closing weeks of 2020, however, the BAME community turned out unsurprisingly to be the most resistant to or at least hesitant in taking the vaccine. While older members of these communities were more likely than younger ones to want the vaccine (when it would be made available), the skewing of the hesitation was clear, as 71.8 per cent of the Black community and 42.3 per cent of the Pakistani/Bangladeshi community showed hesitancy. When asked, they expressed fear of the unknown future effects of the vaccine.[59] Not medical history, not Tuskegee, not even systemic racism, but rather the very same variable that moved a rather high percentage of American healthcare workers (39 per cent) to refuse vaccination at the same moment.[60] Education and gender did play a role in Britain, but community identity, as self-defined 'nations' within a 'nation', was most important, as the anxiety had become part of their symbolic regimen.

While the messages are clear, what remains unclear and often confusing is who exactly is covered by the abbreviation BAME. In May 2020 a study undertaken by the Royal College of Psychiatrists (RCPsych) noted there are two parallel yet different terms used in Britain for individuals from various ethnic backgrounds other than White: one is BAME, the acronym for Black, Asian and Minority Ethnic; the other is BME, which stands for Black and Minority Ethnic. While a 2019 analysis by the NHS Trust, 'Workforce Race Equality Standard', used the term BME, the RCPsych study opted for the term BAME, even though the authors also recognize that 'within the BAME groups, there are some groups which may be more at risk than others.'[61] Or at least in different ways and to different degrees. Another review published by Public Health England on disparities in the risk and outcomes of COVID-19 complicated the matter even further. While the review used the term BAME, under the section on ethnicity being a contributing factor to a higher risk of death, after sex, age, level of deprivation and region, it also states:

> people of Bangladeshi ethnicity had around twice the risk
> of death than people of White British ethnicity. People of

Chinese, Indian, Pakistani, Other Asian, Black Caribbean and Other Black ethnicity had between 10 and 50% higher risk of death when compared to White British . . . These analyses did not account for the effect of occupation, comorbidities or obesity.[62]

If the very terms for impacted minority groups are contested, it is also the case that when we turn to how the constituent elements are imagined, we see radically different ideas of how these groups respond to their victim status. An earlier study of the 2007 Citizenship Survey of 120 BAME members, spanning different ages, genders and social economic groups as well as geographic areas, suggested that perceptions of racial discrimination among BAME minority groups defined as 'victims' varied widely. 'Perceptions of racial discrimination', according to the study, 'were found to be an outcome of the interaction between "psychosocial" factors, on the one hand, and service-specific factors, on the other.' It continued that

The drivers of perceptions of racial discrimination in public services are many and complex. Some precede any personal contact with services, others are outcomes of direct experiences. Some are based exclusively on personal experiences; others draw on formal knowledge and the media. Some are specific to certain services, others are cross-cutting. Some are more amenable to change through policy, others are not (at least in the short to medium term). Some are important to 'high' discrimination respondents, others matter more to 'medium' or 'low' discrimination respondents. For all these reasons, it is not possible to simply rank the drivers of perceptions of racial discrimination and to determine which are the 'most influential' ones overall. Nor is it possible to identify a simple solution to improve everyone's perceptions of racial discrimination. Change will necessarily be slow and uneven.[63]

Here we can add one further caveat about the fallacy of the 'ranking of prejudice' during the pandemic. Excluded or marginalized minorities covered by the acronym BAME were seen to be coterminous with risk for infection in Britain. This seems evident when the clear statistical evidence is examined; indeed, each category reinforces the other. But in Britain, the question of who is 'ethnic' or an 'ethnic minority' already predisposes this statistical correlation. The comedian and social commentator David Baddiel, in his recent popular book, *Jews Don't Count* (2020), points out that Jews do not seem to be considered an ethnic minority in Britain in the public's mind (or, we can add, in such discussions of the pandemic as those we have noted above). As he notes, 'most people . . . might not actively exclude Jews [from BAME], once someone like me points out to them that Jews are actually an ethnic minority, who get discriminated against and suffer racism.'[64] As we have discussed in Chapter Three, Jews, at least ultra-Orthodox Jews in Britain, analogous to those categories listed under BAME, also have a very much higher rate of morbidity and mortality than the general population from the novel coronavirus, yet are not seen as having the same risk factors. Baddiel stresses that Jews do not 'benefit' from positive discrimination (affirmative action, in American terms) because their status as a discriminated-against ethnic minority is invisible.[65] Indeed, the notion that they should, he writes, seems odd, as they are seen, following the antisemitic stereotype, as wealthy (read: miserly), intelligent (read: shrewd) and White. The latter, of course, is consistently denied by anti-semites, who see the Jews' assumption of Whiteness or even 'White privilege' as part of their pernicious racial ability to mimic other groups to those groups' detriment.[66] They are also put into a separate category when it comes to discussions of COVID-19: they are 'to blame' rather than 'innocent victims'. Here, per-haps, we should cite George Bernard Shaw's caustic comment concerning Alfred Doolittle (*nomen est omen*) in his *Pygmalion* (1913). Doolittle notes that he is a member of the 'undeserving poor', while all the benefits go to the so-called 'deserving poor' because of 'middle-class morality'. Yet his needs are not lesser than theirs; indeed, in many ways they are greater, as he needs to support his pleasures, which they reject. We know well that the line drawn between those to blame and those to pity is a reflex of the observer, not an objective evaluation of the one who is ill. Indeed, the recent Conservative government's Commission on Race and Ethnic Disparities report, as we have noted, seems to locate the blame for the greater health disparity of BAME people squarely on the shoulders of the dead and the dying. All surveys and scientific as well as popular discussions of COVID-19 separate these two categories and deal with them as mutually exclusive. This is true in the United States as well as in Britain. Now, British law is crystal clear when it comes to defining minorities. Jews are covered by the Race Relations Act of 1965 (and then the expanded, revised law of 1976, which is in turn broadened by the Equality Act of 2010), which prohibits discrimination on 'grounds of colour, race, or ethnic or national origins'. Note that they are not the subject of the law because of their religious identity but are included as part of an ethnic or racial definition. This formulation was strongly supported by the Jewish Board of Deputies when the law was being promulgated to answer the violence aimed at the rising number of immigrants from the former British colonies in South Asia and the Caribbean. Jews are legally BAME but are not functionally understood as such. To understand how transparent such exclusion is in contemporary Britain dealing with COVID-19, imagine defining an ethnic minority in London, Manchester or Liverpool in 1890 or, indeed in 1920. Suddenly the 'minority ethnic' communities defined by prejudice, discrimination and economic marginality would of course include Jews, then defined by the influx of (Eastern European) Jews, but also the (Catholic) Irish and the (Southern) Italians. All groups, of course, with extraordinary exposure to the risks of illness and poverty now understood as intrinsic to BAME communities. As we have said repeatedly: language matters.

Nevertheless, in the wake of George Floyd's death in the United States, the British have been reminded over and again that 'Racism is a British issue.' Black Britons have been persuaded never to forget the historical racism in 'racist Britain':

> Excusing or downplaying British racism with comparisons to the U.S. is a bad habit with a long history. It began in 1807, with the abolition of the slave trade and picked up steam three decades later with the end of British slavery, twin events that marked the beginning of 200 years of moral posturing and historical amnesia. The Victorian readers who rightly wept over *Uncle Tom's Cabin*, for example, conveniently forgot which nation had carried his ancestors into slavery and didn't dwell on the fact that most of the cotton produced by American slaves like him was shipped to Liverpool. For two centuries, we have deployed American racism as a distraction. It's as if we find it easier

to recognise American forms of racism than we do our own home-grown varieties. Convenient, as pointing fingers is always more comforting than looking in the mirror.

This from David Olusoga, the British public historian and media commentator.[67]

Inspired by Black Lives Matter, protests against British racism swept across the UK, and consequently the use of the term BAME has grown in prominence. The racial discrimination that BAME communities continue to suffer in contemporary Britain is evidenced by the high COVID-19-related mortality and morbidity among members of such groups. Partly reacting to the media coverage of BAME and COVID-19, however, in an interview with the BBC, the British comedian Eshaan Akbar, of half Bangladeshi and half Pakistani parentage, rejected the term 'BAME' outright:

> I hate the term 'BAME,' 'people of colour,' all these labels, they don't define me . . . During the pandemic, in the news all I could hear was the 'BAME community' were the most affected by the illness but this was misleading . . . During the Black Lives Matter protests, 'BAME' popped up yet again . . . But many Muslim Asians felt that issues happening in their community were being ignored . . . The only thing I know we definitely have in common with other people in the 'BAME' group is that we all have really good food.[68]

If for Eshaan it is good food that links BAME communities together, a long-term study by a group of geneticists at Queen Mary University of London suggests that poor health is also a factor that unites Asian communities, particularly South Asian communities, across different parts of the UK, from East London to Bradford. (We can note that 'South Asia' is a multi-ethnic, multi-religious, multicultural sub-continent, but in the UK these different ethnic groups are lumped together as one under the label 'South Asian'. Clearly nineteenth-century colonial ethno-racial categories are still very much alive in twenty-first-century multicultural and multi-ethnic Britain.) According to the study, these communities have descended 'from two ancestral human populations'. They have inherited 'particular' genes that 'can contribute to certain diseases' such as coronary heart disease (CHD).[69] In addition to their particular genes inherited from those distant ancestors, Dr Sandy Gupta, a consultant cardiologist previously at Whipps Cross and St Bartholomew's Hospital who is also of South Asian heritage, pointed to these communities' shared taste for 'unhealthy' food. According to him, this can lead to serious health risks.[70] During the current pandemic, while blaming the South Asians for the high rate of COVID-19, Lord Bethell told the House of Lords in a recent debate on tackling obesity that 'It is true that many people from rural communities in the subcontinent bring with them eating habits that are simply not appropriate for modern life. We have seen that in COVID, where some of the most challenging incidents of COVID have been in communities where there is a high level of people from the subcontinent, whose eating habits, frankly, have left them in no good state to fight this horrible disease.'[71] This was clearly analogous to the debates in the United States about excess weight in the African American community resulting from 'slave' eating practices. The attendant risk for obesity and high blood pressure was traced to these patterns of consumption. While such factors as eating practices were vital in these discussions up to 2020, they have virtually vanished in the age of COVID-19, even though the mounting evidence that obesity (and resultant type

2 diabetes) is a major risk factor has been stressed for the entire (overweight) American population.[72] Again, food can be viewed as a source of pleasure or danger, depending who is speaking, and what purpose is served.

Not only do researchers' perceptions of risk differ, depending on which dataset is used for analysis, but the conclusions they draw from them also vary substantially. A joint study by a group of researchers from Queen Mary University London, the NHS Trust and the University of Oxford using the data supplied by UK Biobank (UKB) pointed to the limitations of the dataset, because the very categories employed, such as age range, ethnic variations, wider social, economic and behavioural factors, were not nuanced enough to capture clear causation. They drew the conclusion that 'factors which underlie ethnic differences in COVID-19 may not be easily captured' and that the 'ethnicity differential pattern of COVID-19 is not adequately explained by variations in cardiometabolic factors, 25(OH)-vitamin D levels, socio-economic or behavioural factors'. Hence, 'aggregating all BAME populations may overlook important differences between ethnicities; studies in samples with greater ethnic diversity are needed.'[73] Nevertheless, the study agrees with the 'growing reports of higher risk of severe COVID-19 in men and BAME populations'. It is not only the growing number of cases that points to the greater risk to BAME communities of COVID-19; as in the United States the litmus test for the source of community disquiet seems to be the willingness of these groups to undertake vaccination or, in earlier moments, to become a subject for vaccine field tests.[74] Lumped together because of poverty, family structure, geography and racial stereotyping, these groups are disaggregated when this litmus test is applied. After the first two mRNA vaccines were announced, 76 per cent of the general

UK population were willing to be vaccinated if advised to by a health professional, according to polling for the Royal Society for Public Health (RSPH). On the contrary, only 57 per cent of BAME individuals as a collective would, but if this were disaggregated, only 55 per cent of Asian ancestry would take the vaccine.[75] The rationales given are familiar. For the Asian community, implicitly defined as either Muslim or Hindu even though there are Asian Christians, Sikhs, Parsees and Jews present in the UK, it is the idea that the content is not acceptable, not the process. Earlier the NHS had distributed childhood immunizations throughout Britain that contained pork gelatin as a stabilizer and did not provide any that did not. As a Muslim physician notes, 'We are paying the price for that now because people are saying "Oh, vaccines have gelatin," or they are just not interested in listening to us.'[76] As we noted earlier, among ultra-Orthodox Jews this seems to be a legend made flesh by the 2019 measles epidemic in New York City and reinformed by COVID-19. Yet the initial mRNA vaccines are free of such elements. The variable present here, given the contested nature of these vaccines, is the varied set of symbols concerning health and illness ascribed to the disparate religious communities within 'BAME'. For even in Muslim-majority countries impacted by such claims (Afghanistan, Malaysia, Pakistan) about the unavailability of halal-certified vaccines, 'in cases of dire (Arabic language termed as *dorurah*) and necessary circumstances which are recognized by the Islamic law (Shariah law), necessity overrules prohibitions. In circumstances where no available halal sources or options are effective in treating the disease, the *hukm* becomes permissible (termed *harus* in Arabic), for instance in vaccination.'[77] One can note that an analogous path of argument is to be found among Jewish religious leaders.[78] Indeed, as we have discussed above and as medical anthropologist Ben Kasstan has observed, anti-vaxxers in the Haredi community often avoided religious opinions concerning vaccines in the past as they assumed that the religious authorities would advocate for immunization.[79] Recently, even this generalization, as he has noted, has come under the influence of global anti-vaxxing propaganda.[80] Thus the problem has to do with self-definition shaped by the increased importance of diasporic evocation of local traditions, rather than absolute, 'universal' religious prohibitions.

As for Black communities in Britain, the search for the causes of their resistance falls back on hoary arguments about African American communities. When in March 2020 the trials for the proposed vaccines were held, the public consensus claimed that 'among black and minority ethnic (BAME) patients, distrust in research and medical professionals was also a common reason given for not wanting to participate.' Dr Peter Knapp from the Department of Health Sciences at the University of York and the Hull York Medical School further observed that 'Lack of trust was also identified as a common barrier for minority ethnic patients around the world – perhaps a legacy of major historical violations of ethical standards in cases like the Tuskegee syphilis experiment.'[81] Now, one can claim that the legacy of these cases, exemplified by the Tuskegee Experiment, has shaped African American attitudes as they became part of a late twentieth-century discourse about race and medicine, but there seems to be little evidence of analogous cases in British medicine. One needs to note that this is a shift in argument responding to the American model in the media. Earlier studies of vaccine resistance as shown in a 2017 retrospective literature review saw cultural factors ('namely religion, upbringing and migration, and language') as impacting parents' choice to immunize their children. The central question was 'whether immunisations were permitted or culturally acceptable'. Only then did 'perceived biological differences [affect] decision-making and demand for information'.[82] Assumed historical memory and culture evidently played no role in this set of choices in 2016. This is not to say that prior to 2020 in the NHS (and the ongoing idiosyncrasies of the so-called 'postcode lottery') minorities were not marginalized, poorly serviced and the object of both scorn and anxiety. How can we expect these disadvantaged groups to be enthusiastic about the vaccine when they lack opportunity and social capability, and are not prioritized for the vaccination?[83] How can we expect them to participate in any public health project when the society around them has continued to view them as being 'sick' or 'unhealthy'? But Tuskegee now has become a touchstone for all the misdeeds of allopathic medical research. After the vaccines were approved, little changed in the rationale.

The official statements of Jonathan Van-Tam, one of the UK government's scientific advisers, when asked about the special status of the Black community as a priority for vaccination noted 'that people with underlying medical conditions were already prioritized, and many BAME people would fall into that category, but there was no plan for ethnicity alone to be a criterion'. Yet these groups, however defined, are most at risk, according to virtually every authority who has written about it. Van-Tam's odd circumlocution was explained in the press by the 'the malign spectre of history and the record of the United States, in particular, of having exploited black people for medical trials. The notorious Tuskegee syphilis study, which lasted from the 1930s into the 1970s and was the subject of an apology from President Bill Clinton, is perhaps the most notorious example.'[84] Indeed the very claim that BAME groups as a collective are particularly vulnerable to COVID-19 comes to be part of this rationale, as Professor Sophie Harman, who specializes in the politics of global health at Queen Mary University of London, observes: 'Would you trust a government that accepts you're more likely to die of COVID-19 than your white neighbours and does nothing very much about it? Vaccine hesitancy risks a double tragedy: racial inequality in deaths from Covid-19 and potential racial inequality in vaccine uptake.'[85] The culture of trust needs to be cultivated, and the way to begin such a process is to move away from narratives of resistance of the vulnerable groups and the salvation offered by the state authorities and medical 'heroes'. COVID-19 has revealed two types of health disparities: the first exists among those who are actually at greater risk as defined by their statistical rate of morbidity and mortality; the second, by the symbolic register within (and about) these groups concerning both the experience of anxiety, fear and vulnerability and the assumptions that such groups are simultaneously placing others at risk. Such communities are already vulnerable socially and economically. COVID-19 has just added another challenge to their fragility or the struggle for survival of their members.

Such disparities have been uniformly laid at the feet of economic factors as well as group identity. But during the second wave of the pandemic, prior to the advent of the broadly successful vaccine campaign at the end of 2020, the differences between groups were shown to have been ameliorated. At that point the category of BAME seemed to splinter as a useful public health indicator. One published study recently suggests that in the second wave of infections in the UK, while the disparities remained more pronounced in people of South Asian ethnicity, particularly those from Pakistani and Bangladeshi heritages, compared to people from other ethnic groups, the members of those groups were more likely to reside in deprived areas, in large households and in multigenerational families. The same study also suggested that in the second wave, people from Black ethnic groups were no longer at any greater risk of COVID-19 mortality compared to those of White British ethnicity.[86]

The truth of these claims can be seen in the extraordinary fact that, in the United States, as vaccine rollouts took place in December 2020 and January 2021, minorities, Black, Latinx and Indigenous communities had massively lower rates of vaccination than White communities of all economic levels, often two to three times lower.[87] We could expect such vaccine hesitancy, to use the now fashionable term, to stem from the often repeated and quite accurate mantra that these communities have been the target of medical abuse in the past. Yet the reality is that the basic reason is not 'hesitancy' but inaccessibility. Vaccines had been shipped to medical centres, to pharmacies, to mass vaccination sites: all these were inaccessible to minority communities. To no one's surprise, such structures exist primarily in White, middle-class communities or are accessible only by car, not the radically reduced urban public transportation of the pandemic. In Washington, DC, where one of the authors of this book lives, when the meagre numbers of vaccines made available to the community were announced, middle-class White patients suddenly began to show up for vaccination in the few private and public health clinics in primarily Black, working-class neighbourhoods. Those getting vaccinated had easier access to computers, iPhones and cars, while the locals, without these resources, missed out – not because they purposefully avoided vaccination but because they simply could not get into the virtual queue for it. After this became apparent, the city required individuals to register only in their local zip codes to get their vaccines locally, and the primarily middle-class White zip codes were excluded.[88] This was true across the United States: in Miami, minorities were severely underrepresented in vaccinations even though they were overrepresented in the numbers of cases, hospitalizations and deaths. By early February 2021 only 7 per cent of the recipients of vaccines in Miami were Black, even though this community comprises nearly 17 per cent of the city's population and its death rate is more than 60 per cent higher than that of Whites. One can note that as of the end of January the vaccine rollout in the United States was chaotic and haphazard because of the total lack of planning by the Trump administration, which had been concerned only with the delivery of vaccine to the states, not the actual 'shots in arms', the immunization of individuals in myriad geographic and symbolic communities. In the UK the situation concerning vaccine availability had been much better than this after the beginning of 2021, even though the lack of planning under Boris Johnson over the course of the pandemic led to extraordinarily high rates of morbidity and mortality in the country and even greater losses in BAME communities. About half of those in these minority communities, at least at the rollout, were opting to not be vaccinated.[89] Most Blacks (29 per cent) stated that their concern was about mass testing to assure the safety of the vaccine; most South Asians worried about potential side effects. History seems to have played no measurable factor in any of the surveys undertaken in either the United Kingdom or the United States, even though interpreters of the data may read this into their analysis. And this heightened anxiety dissipates over time as the simple fact that people you know have had the vaccine mitigates fear, as a recent Press Ganey survey has shown. Even among African Americans in the United States, who had the lowest rate of desire to be vaccinated, the key to acceptance was provider advice within the community, which negated most distrust about the vaccine.[90] Certainly history, especially popular history such as the repeated account of the Tuskegee Experiment, as the Press Ganey survey noted, played a role in the initial hesitation: 'I remember Tuskegee. The government was not kind toward the Black American male! I don't trust the government and you can't blame me!!'[91] Yet the reality is that the structural racism that made it harder for all minorities in the United States and UK to access the vaccine was at the core of any discrepancies. As in the case of the city of Leicester in the UK, arguably the city with highest portion of people of South Asian ethnicities and with some of the highest rates of morbidity and mortality during the current pandemic, once the initial hurdles were overcome, suddenly, with this level playing field, all communities accessed the vaccines in more or less equal numbers.[92]

5

TRUMP AS SYMBOL: ANGER WITHIN AND AGAINST 'WHITE' COMMUNITIES

On 8 October 2020, a Thursday teeming with events leading up to the 3 November presidential election in the United States, thirteen people were charged by the FBI and Michigan state authorities with participating in a plot to kidnap, try and execute the state of Michigan's Democratic governor, Gretchen Whitmer. They had called her a 'tyrant' because of her attempts to control the pandemic. (A further individual was added to the federal and state charges later.) At least three of the men accused, who styled themselves the 'Wolverine Watchmen', had participated on 30 April in the occupation of the Michigan State Capitol in Lansing, wearing body armour and carrying pistols and long guns.[1] The Republican-dominated legislature, opened by the Senate majority leader, a Republican, singing the Protestant hymn 'It Is Well with My Soul', had declared that Whitmer's attempt to limit the spread of COVID-19 was an 'overreach' and illegal. The breaching of the Michigan state house to contest violently the public health measures put in place to combat the pandemic on 30 April 2020, and the subsequent threats to try and execute the governor as well as occupy the legislature, were rehearsals for the 6 January 2021 storming of the Capitol in Washington, DC. Six of the Trump supporters who invaded the Lansing legislature were arrested after the insurrection in Washington for having overrun the Capitol. The initial protest was organized by Meshawn Maddock, who later filled nineteen buses with demonstrators to protest in Washington. He was subsequently elected co-chair of the Michigan Republican Party.[2] The Washington protest had been attended and planned by many of the same groups with precisely the same intent: to nullify lawful state activities through armed force, in this case the November election, by seizing and, if the gallows erected on the Capitol grounds was any indication, executing the culprits, including the Vice-President of the United States, their putative ally in all things and the head of the federal Coronavirus Task Force.

'Anti-lockdown' had morphed into 'anti-electoral fraud'. And an overwhelming number of the participants in the 6 January insurrection had been involved in loud and often violent opposition to state-wide mandates issued to help mitigate the spread of the virus, an opposition led and echoed by the then president. Trump's wilful public denial of the severity of the pandemic early on and his regular minimization of it, even as hundreds of thousands died, was the message heard by the rioters. Profiles of those who were at the demonstration illustrated this tight connection of public disorder to pandemic grievances of all sorts. Thus Pete Harding, a 47-year-old construction worker from upstate New York, had earlier been arrested for refusing to leave a liquor store when asked to wear a mask. He subsequently voted for Trump as a statement against pandemic mandates, saying at the time, 'We know that if Biden-Harris was going to get into office, they've said they're going to make the lockdowns mandatory and mask-wearing mandatory across the country.' He was at the Capitol and joined the mob: 'I started to see everybody going up the stairs at that point, and I decided I needed to be up there.'[3] All this was of a piece. The support of the Republican members of the House and Senate, who instigated the insurrection through their unprincipled support of the false claim of election fraud, had been prefigured by the Michigan representatives and judges months earlier.

After the armed invasion of the Michigan legislature, the Republican-dominated Michigan Supreme Court overturned the governor's attempts to control what came to be a massive spike in infection through her power to take emergency action based on laws passed in the 1940s. The public's health was less vital to the public, the courts intimated, than the ability of the state legislature to control the governor's actions. Katherine Henry, the attorney who won the case advocating for the freedom to infect oneself and others, advised citizens,

> That means burn your masks right now if you didn't already. Open your gym, and movie theatre and open whatever business you have. Go on and frequent whatever business you would like to go to, if you have a church that's limited your services because of how you're reading the EOS, forget that. All of those executive orders, based on COVID-19 circumstances, from 2020, they're out, they're gone, they're done.[4]

This, one can add, in anticipation of the deadly spikes of infection in the autumn and winter of 2020, which hit Michiganders, now able to have their unfettered freedom to die and kill others, unmasked, undistanced, unprepared. And it worked. By 1 January 2021 one of every 1,000 Michiganders was dead from COVID-19, the highest death rate in the state since 1936. Freedom has its consequences.

Such a position, including that expressed by the Michigan Supreme Court, which holds individual 'freedom', here a euphemism for licence, higher than the common good, ignored the obvious claims in blackletter law holding that the public's health should be the most important factor in times of pandemic, whether in terms of economic closure or quarantine. It is 'freedom from' in the Hobbesian use of 'liberty', meaning the unfettered action of human beings living in what he imagined to be a state of nature. This is understood by him as the absence of interference in any of one's activities (to use Isaiah Berlin's famous definition of negative 'freedom from' in his 1958 lecture on 'Two Concepts of Liberty'[5]). But true freedom demands in the end an accountability to the collective, freedom limited in order to substantially protect those in your world from harm, if at all possible. Thomas Hobbes saw that by each subsuming themselves to the power of the political community they are rescued from the terrors of such 'liberty', where 'there is perpetual war of every man against his neighbor; no inheritance to transmit to the son, nor to expect from the father; no propriety of goods or lands; no security.'[6] And we can add random exposure to death and social displacement from plague, something with which Hobbes would have been well acquainted, as friends and patrons had died of it. Remember Thomas Hobbes was the first English translator of Thucydides' *History of the Peloponnesian War* (1629), with its account of the chaos following the Athenian plague that was blamed on the Ethiopians. And his *Leviathan or The Matter, Forme and Power of a Commonwealth Ecclesiasticall and Civil* (1651) is a work that brings this fear of social collapse in social chaos to the fore. Abraham Bosse's frontispiece of Hobbes's *Leviathan* includes, among other figures, two plague doctors wearing full PPE (at least for the seventeenth century), including beaked masks, walking the streets of an abandoned cityscape.[7] The individual more or less voluntarily submits to the fear of the law and to the terror of the 'public sword' to avoid such worlds.[8]

Sir William Blackstone's eighteenth-century commentary on British jurisprudence, *Commentaries on the Laws of England* (1765–9), annotating the 1603 law on plague under James I, summarizes that fear of the 'public sword':

> any person infected with the plague, or dwelling in any infected house, he commanded by the mayor or constable, or other head officer of his town or vill, to keep his house, and shall venture to disobey it; he may be enforced, by the watchmen appointed on such melancholy occasions, to obey such necessary command: and, if any hurt ensue by such enforcement, the watchmen are thereby indemnified. And farther, if such person of commanded to confine himself goes abroad, and converses in company, if he has no plague sore upon him, he shall be punished as a vagabond by whipping, and be bound to his good behaviour: but, if he has any infectious sore upon him uncured, he then shall be guilty of felony.[9]

While we would no longer advocate public whipping for such breaches of health conventions, the notion that the state had the primary ability to at least attempt to control the spread of disease was well established even before more modern views of the dangers of infectious diseases to the public's health. One can acknowledge that state interventions will never be invincible against an infectious pathogen, but the absence of any such enforceable state or collective actions almost guarantees its spread. What Blackstone and indeed most legal systems recognize is that the state has an interest in preserving the overall health of its citizens. Blackstone's mid-eighteenth-century views had a formative influence on the writing of the American

Constitution in 1787 and subsequent legal theory and practice. Among the absolute rights he advocated were 'personal security' that assures the enjoyment of 'life' and 'health'. American constitutional law holds that the states may pass and enforce laws that are intended to control the spread and eradication of epidemics.[10] In constituting the symbolic register for the national community, health (here defined as combating disease) is an absolute defining aspect of community identity.[11] Thomas Hobbes's notion of the obligation of the state to correct for the self-destructive actions of individuals overrules John Locke's demand for individual liberty. Under such circumstances, the attempts of thinkers such as Amitai Etzioni in the 1990s to create a so-called responsive communitarianism, which gives equal weight to the common good and the idea of individual rights, must fail.

Cass R. Sunstein and Adrian Vermeule have recently made a version of our argument about the necessity of a Hobbesian perspective for a proactive state in their defence of the administrative state, labelling this as '*the* morality of administrative law'.[12] They also consider the question of what constitutes a moral legal system and conclude that legal systems such as those of the Nazis are by definition not legal systems at all.[13] Here we might say that those that manipulate a legal system for perverse aims, such as putting individuals at risk of infection in the name of 'freedom', are equally not legal systems. Sunstein and Vermeule ask:

> those who support the administrative state deny that it is a threat to liberty, properly understood. Consider some of the actual activities of that state. Would people be freer without child labor laws? . . . Without protection against

pandemics? Some defenders of the administrative state argue that it is not only constitutionally permissible, but also in some sense mandatory, if the goal is to carry into execution the promises of the constitutional scheme.[14]

Blackstone would have been delighted.

History Again on the Block

The earlier demonstration against the state's imposition of measures to control the pandemic in Lansing brought out signs decorated with swastikas that read 'Heil Whitmer!' And one of its leaders, Karl Manke, a barber raised in a German-speaking Lutheran home, commented on the demonstrations against 'government overreach': 'They would trade their liberty for security . . . Because the Nazis told them, "Get in these cattle cars, and we're gonna take you to a nice, safe place. Just get in."' In 2014 Manke had also published a novel, *Age of Shame*, about a Jewish victim of the Holocaust and a German victim of ethnic cleansing in post-war Eastern Europe. The linkage between the idea that American conservatives suffered (and suffer) as victims of the state and the predations of the Nazis is, as we have seen over and over again, a theme during the pandemic. Manke's novel recreates a parallel between the systematic extirpation of the Jews and the expulsion of ethnic Germans. This correspondence created an equivalence between 'victims' favoured by the revanchist circles of German refugees from Eastern Europe in West Germany (*Vertriebenenverbände*) from the 1950s to the '80s. Everyone here is a victim of an oppressive regime. When he presented a copy to a reporter interviewing him, 'Manke wrote, "History unheeded is history repeated."'[15] By now George Santayana's formulation of the danger of forgetting history (rooted in his Hegelian belief that 'savages' had none, as we discussed in the prior chapter) had become a ubiquitous Internet meme, and, it seems, a persistent feature of public debates about COVID-19.

On 17 April 2020 the then president of the United States, Donald Trump, tweeted to his followers to 'LIBERATE MICHIGAN' from the person he dismissively called 'that woman in Michigan'. The members of the Wolverine Watchmen heard it as a rallying call, reinforcing their plan to kill Whitmer and burn down the State Capitol (which was dominated by Republicans). Their anti-government ideology embraced the notion that 'A well-armed citizenry is the best form of Homeland Security and can better deter crime, invasion, terrorism, and tyranny.'[16] It was Trump, through his own ambiguities concerning such groups, who had come to serve as a single symbolic reference for all the 'antis' during the pandemic: anti-vaccine, anti-public health measures, anti-science, anti-masking, anti-state authority (unless the authority is ambiguous or his own).[17] Trump's statement about vigilantes (regarding the Proud Boys, another so-called militia) in his first debate with Joe Biden, that they should 'stand back and stand by', and then his subsequent attempt to walk this back, is indicative of this purposeful ambiguity.[18]

Trump's function as a symbolic reference for the widest range of claims about the pandemic is central to any understanding of the attachment of blame and its denial among White conservative communities. 'His base has been primed to believe conspiracies and disbelieve in official accounts,' commented Joan Donovan, a disinformation expert at Harvard University. 'The skepticism that allows him to draw in these communities is the same skepticism that they are bringing to this world historic moment.'[19] We would amend this view to note that Trump's ideological followers believe that his amorphous views represent their collective symbolic register, even if it also contradicts other supporters' worldviews. This belief has been regularly reinforced by Trump's funnelling such beliefs through simply retweeting them. By 6 January 2021 that was clearly not enough, as he held a rally in front of the White House, again decrying that the election had been stolen from him and his followers and urging them

> to walk down [to the Capitol] and I'll be there with you. We're going to walk down. We're going to walk down any one you want, but I think right here. We're going walk down to the Capitol, and we're going to cheer on our brave senators, and congressmen and women. We're probably not going to be cheering so much for some of them because you'll never take back our country with weakness. You have to show strength, and you have to be strong.[20]

Egged on, they marched and invaded the Capitol. The speech, so focused on his own victim status, mentioned neither the explosion of cases across the country nor the mangled rollout of the vaccines. As Justice Oliver Wendell Holmes Jr observed in 1919 in *Abrams v. United States* (250 U.S. 616), 'falsely shouting "fire" in a theater and causing a panic' is not an act blessed by the First Amendment of the American Constitution and its guarantee of the freedom of speech from government interference.[21] The irony is that the theatre was actually on fire, the pandemic had filled hospitals across the country and the death rate exceeded that of the worst days of the prior spring, but Trump was so focused on 'falsely shouting' that the election had been stolen that he, unmasked, and the mainly unmasked crowds at his rally, seemed to be oblivious of COVID-19. Some even believed that they were invulnerable and Trump's almost 'heroic' recovery from the novel coronavirus was their proof. The rhetoric of the 'stolen' election invoked by Trump was psychologically very powerful for these White supporters. Many of them truly believe, cognitively, that their misfortunes and miseries are the result of being 'robbed'. The culprits were either the Chinese or illegal immigrants or Jewish plutocrats or the BLM mob, or all of them in concert, and Trump was the white knight in shining armour who would help them get back what was truly theirs. Indeed, all these groups, over the course of the year, had been blamed for spreading the virus, whether by purposely developing it in a laboratory in Wuhan (according to Trump's Secretary of State Mike Pompeo and his CDC Director Robert Redfield) or by smuggling their infected bodies across the Southern border (according to the Governor of Texas, Greg Abbott) or by George Soros and the Rothschilds creating a pandemic to control the world economy, never mind Bill Gates and high tech developing a vaccine to place a microchip in your brain![22] Trump's lies became their absolute truths and, for those who subscribe to QAnon and other conspiracy theories, an intrinsic part of their ideology. One can note that a number of sources have been tabulating his 'lies' in the multiple of tens of thousands.[23] By the end of his term in office he had lied, misspoken, misdirected and obfuscated 30,573 times, over fifty a day.[24] One needs to see such public utterances as megaphones for the belief systems of the various collectives that have defined Trump as their common referent.

All these groups who identified with Trump's rhetoric saw themselves as 'victims', and victimhood became the rhetoric through which they placed the blame for the pandemic, as well as everything else they perceived as violating their symbolic self-definitions, no matter how contradictory. The political scientists Miles T. Armaly and Adam M. Enders distinguish between those who presented as 'egocentric (i.e., "I am the victim because I deserve more than I get") or systemic (i.e., "I am the victim because the system is rigged against me").'[25] While they argue that these are two distinct aspects of identification, they saw, and the realities of 6 January 2021 bore them out, that both of them were quite independent of any objective correlatives, such as the psychological, economic or social locations of the participant. That is, their perception of the world was located in the symbolic realm, rather than in one of lived experience. Armaly and Enders elaborate:

> Victimhood is a central theme of modern political messaging. For instance, a Republican strategist observed, 'At a Trump rally, central to the show is the idea of shared victimization . . . Trump revels in it, has consistently portrayed himself as a victim of the media and of his political opponents . . .'. However, if you consider Trump's demographic characteristics (white and male) and his successes (in terms of wealth and being president), he is not a victim by any serious societal standard. While Trump's supporters may, to varying degrees, be victims of certain social and political circumstances, the rallies at which the president is reveling in their shared victimhood are direct consequences of at least their recent political successes.

Symbols matter and Armaly and Enders conclude that 'perceived victimhood is neither a mere reflection of "true" victim status or previously identified personality traits, nor a post hoc justification for maintaining the status quo. Instead, it cuts across the social and political hierarchy.' But they maintain that

'Victimhood, in some form, is related to anti-establishment attitudes, political efficacy, personality traits, racial attitudes, and support for particular political candidates.' And we can add to this list 'White privilege'.

At this point we want to make a historical parallel without attempting to be overly simplistic, as was the Michigan demonstrator Karl Manke: no, history does not repeat itself, for good or for ill. But there are overall functions inherent in the symbolic construction of all imagined communities which allow us to understand the focus and motivation of those who chose Donald Trump as their symbolic referent in now seeing themselves as the 'victims' of a COVID-19 'conspiracy', not the actual disease – which many still deny exists. By the use of ambiguity all the way through his term of office, but especially in his public persona during the pandemic, Trump has functioned as a central element in the symbolic register of a very wide range of ideological positions in which he is the overlapping moment in a complex Venn diagram. When in response to the demonstrations in August 2017 in Charlottesville, Virginia, that left one person dead and many wounded, he stated, 'You had some very bad people in that group, but you also had people that were very fine people, on both sides,' this was a way of appeasing groups who may have taken umbrage to his earlier comments that outright condemned right-wing racism. The ambiguity was clearly intended.[26]

After being labelled 'the invisible politician' following his release from Landsberg prison in 1924, Adolf Hitler had precisely that same function as the focus of competing ideological worldviews in the 1920s and '30s.[27] We know that the history of Nazism has long served as a quarry for historical analogies in the post-war period. Whenever a political debate or an international crisis reaches fever pitch, someone is (and was) likely to deploy a Nazi analogy. Indeed, Godwin's Law states that the longer an online exchange continues, the greater the chance that Hitler, the Nazis or the Third Reich will be invoked. Major political figures around the world have been routinely compared to Nazi leaders in order to tarnish their reputation and policies, or to justify a particular course of action. Before the first Iraq War, for instance, George H. W. Bush famously compared Saddam Hussein to Hitler. Circumstances, too, have come in for comparisons: has the United States reached a 'Weimar moment' in view of the sharp political polarization of society? For good or ill, our contemporary political discourse is infused with Nazi analogies, a trend that accelerated with the beginnings of the Trump presidency in 2016.[28] The critical literature on this is clear: such analogues, like evoking Santayana in any context, are fraught with errors. The eminent historian of Nazi Germany Sir Richard Evans is perhaps closest to the mark when he speaks of 'echoes' of the Third Reich rather than parallels to it.[29] The echo we wish to evoke is that both Trump and Hitler served as the focus of a new symbolic register for national and community identity that was composed out of often contradictory registers of various and sundry, sometimes overlapping definitions of community, exploited by both for their own ascension to and maintenance of power. This shaped the symbolic register that eventually labelled the Trumpite tribe as the victims of the pandemic, not necessarily those most at risk from infection, but those most at risk from repression during it.

Trump's expertise in branding is central to this. Indeed, while virtually all his investment and real estate projects were failures, what he managed to sell over time was his brand, a brand fixed in the public sphere by his role as a billionaire on television and reinforced by the leasing of his name to adorn multiple real estate projects and other (often marginally illegal) activities, such as Trump University. In 1991 the American Marketing Association rated Trump as about as impactful a brand name as Bart Simpson.[30] In 2002 Trump's cartoon image was being used by McDonald's to sell dollar Big 'N' Tasty burgers as Bill Lamar, the burger company's vice-president, noted:

> The sandwiches we're offering for a dollar are a great deal, and we chose people like Donald Trump – who know great deals when they see them – to help us make that point in a fun and memorable way. Combining our beloved characters with a high-powered celebrity and adding a little humor really resonates with customers as a way of bringing our value offer to life.[31]

By 2016 this type of franchising of Trump's image was potent enough to be the keystone to his becoming part of the symbolic register for a wider range of American voters, even those who had voted for Barack Obama four years earlier. One can only admire this complexity by noting that in 2020, during the pandemic, the most admired man in the United States was Donald Trump and the most admired woman was Michelle Obama.[32]

Hitler too became a brand, refashioning himself in the 1920s by posing for action photographs while declaiming in the studio of Hans Hoffmann, literally learning how to sell himself to the political public of the day. What he and the nascent National Socialist Party learned early on, and used thereafter, was that they had to sell themselves as the victims, the victims of the Dawes Plan for reparations, of Judeo-Bolshevism, of the November criminals (the Weimar state), of the lying newspapers (*Lügenpresse*), of the conspiracy of the 'Elders of Zion'.

Victimhood, however, did not vanish with political victory after 30 January 1933, with voters across the economic spectrum identifying with 'being victims'. But once established, the 'victims' as well as their newly found enthusiasts began to market themselves. After 1933 controlling Hitler's image became a matter of state. But much of the adulation was spontaneous, or, more precisely, designed to anticipate Hitler's approval. Towns and cities renamed streets and squares after him, poems were composed in his honour (such as the often-republished ode by the head of the Hitler Youth, Baldur von Schirach) and the 'German greeting' of 'Heil Hitler!' became so common that the ss magazine *Das Schwarze Korps* poked fun at the awkward 'German Protestant' and 'German Catholic' greetings. Tailors were instructed in how to cut men's suits to ease the outstretched arm, bakers designed cakes bearing the Führer's name, cafés were renamed after him and shops overflowed with chocolates, picture postcards, china plates, tin horns and photographs bearing his image. Apart from the latter merchandise, which was sold and distributed by the party, the commercial use of Hitler's likeness and name was banned by Joseph Goebbels in May 1933 as 'Führer kitsch'. Controlling the leader's image was a matter of state concern in the 1930s and '40s. Hitler had become a symbol, the value of which had to be maintained through a state that controlled all means of symbolic representation, down to postcards and cakes. With the advent of mass, online social networks, by 2020 it had become more and more possible for an individual (or indeed a collective purporting to be an individual, such as Q) to control their image in not only national but international public spheres.

One needs to understand that the control and manipulation of such images, whether of Donald Trump or Adolf Hitler, emerged not from simple popular acclaim or even fame but from careful marketing. Harold Lasswell noted in 1936 that 'the man of skill in propaganda, witness Lenin, Mussolini and Hitler', could achieve his end in such times of insecurity.[33] In his memoir, Sigmund Freud's Jewish nephew, Edward Bernays, the father of modern advertising psychology ('Reach for a Lucky instead of a Sweet'), commented that at a dinner in New York City in 1933

> Karl von Wiegand, foreign correspondent of the Hearst newspapers, an old hand at interpreting Europe and just returned from Germany, was telling us about Goebbels and his propaganda plans to consolidate Nazi power. Goebbels had shown Wiegand his propaganda library, the best Wiegand had ever seen. Goebbels, said Wiegand, was using my book *Crystallizing Public Opinion* as a basis for his destructive campaign against the Jews of Germany. This shocked me . . . Obviously the attack on the Jews of Germany was no emotional outburst of the Nazis, but a deliberate, planned campaign.[34]

The twentieth century was the first age of marketing that understood the emotional life of the individuals targeted as not only malleable but a potential imagined community. Bernays had in 1928 written a book on propaganda that seems to foretell the employment of the infinitely malleable images of political leaders as part of a symbolic register now defining such a community:

> The conscious and intelligent manipulation of the organized habits and opinions of the masses is an important element in democratic society. Those who manipulate this unseen mechanism of society constitute an invisible

government which is the true ruling power of our country
. . . We are governed, our minds are molded, our tastes
formed, our ideas suggested, largely by men we have never
heard of. This is a logical result of the way in which our
democratic society is organized. Vast numbers of human
beings must cooperate in this manner if they are to live
together as a smoothly functioning society . . . In almost
every act of our daily lives, whether in the sphere of
politics or business, in our social conduct or our ethical
thinking, we are dominated by the relatively small number
of persons . . . who understand the mental processes and
social patterns of the masses. It is they who pull the wires
which control the public mind . . . If we understand the
mechanism and motives of the group mind, is it not possible to control and regiment the masses according to our
will without their knowing about it? The recent practice of
propaganda has proved that it is possible, at least up to a
certain point and within certain limits.[35]

If a national leader is in principle a free-floating signifier that
can be appropriated by the belief systems of those who see him
(or her) as fulfilling or indeed anticipating their best interests
and desires, then that leader becomes symbolic of all that which
is projected onto them and, if the leader does hold strong views,
can use this identification to shape the views of the communities that acknowledge them. The figures represented in Frank
Dikötter's 2019 *How to Be a Dictator: The Cult of Personality in the
Twentieth Century* (Mussolini, Hitler, Stalin, Mao Zedong, Kim
Il-sung, 'Papa Doc' Duvalier, Nicolae Ceauşescu and Mengistu
Haile Mariam) and in Ruth Ben-Ghiat's 2020 *Strongmen: Mussolini
to the Present* (Mussolini, Hitler, Augusto Pinochet, Francisco

Franco, Muammar Qaddafi, Silvio Berlusconi, Mobutu Sese Seko, Viktor Orban, Rodrigo Duterte, Vladimir Putin, Narendra Modi and, centrally, Donald Trump) all fall into this category. Hitler, for example, had only one consistent, indeed obsessive, political view over his entire career: his antisemitism. Every other ideological core of National Socialism mutates over and over again from the 1920s to the 1940s. Indeed, early on there was a general assumption that his anti-Jewish statements were ploys that would also shift once he came into power, a view espoused even by a few very right-wing Jewish politicians of the time, such as Max Samter and Hans-Joachim Schoeps.[36] Trump too held virtually no pronounced ideological views except his xenophobia, which was his brand from the moment he came down the golden escalator at Trump Tower to announce his candidacy in 2015. While anxiety about White status and privilege, defined by xenophobia, certainly marked the response to the wide range of COVID-19 interventions, other symbolic registers were also present, from middle-class, suburban anti-vaxxers to anti-authoritarianism. Not only were virtually all the qualities ascribed to Trump by the forces that coalesced around him during the pandemic projected onto him but he in turn incorporated them, no matter how contrary, into the symbolic register of his own imagined community.

Before we go on to examine the components of the COVID-19 imagined community, let us pause for a minute to ask how massive pandemics in the recent past shaped realpolitik. Kristian S. Blickle of the New York Federal Reserve published a relatively detailed study during the COVID-19 pandemic asking exactly this question. He looked at a set of variables following the destructive pattern of massive deaths during 1918–19 from the Spanish flu on the German home front and the impact on urban voting in the elections up to 1933.[37] Remember that in November 1918 the collapse of the home front was startling to those in Germany and the Austro-Hungarian Empire, who had been led to believe that the advances by their armies were actually winning the war in the West after the Russians (Soviets) had capitulated and the Eastern Front had collapsed. Blickle argues that the simultaneous outbreak of influenza had a magnifying effect on this sense of loss.

> First, we show that areas which experienced a greater relative population decline due to the spread of influenza spend less, per-capita, on their inhabitants in the following decade. This holds especially for spending on amenities more likely to be consumed by the young, for example school funding. Second, influenza deaths of 1918 are correlated with an increase in the share of votes won by right-wing extremists, such as the National Socialist Workers Party (aka, the Nazi Party), in the crucial elections of 1932 and 1933.

That is, the worse the mortality and morbidity during the pandemic, the greater the likelihood that the inhabitants would see the far right (rather than the equally contentious far left, the KPD) as espousing their own state-defining symbolic order. But this is also tied to Blickle's finding that

> the correlation between influenza mortality and the vote share won by right-wing extremists is stronger in regions that had historically blamed minorities, particularly Jews, for medieval plagues. Our findings are possibly tied to the type of victims most directly affected by the virus. Given

that it was disproportionately fatal for young people, the change in demographics may have affected regional attitudes going forward. Moreover, the disease may have fostered a hatred of 'others', as it was perceived to come from abroad.

Which, of course, it did; but not in the ways espoused by the Nazis.[38] That the Black Death is evoked here (and refuted in the manner that we described in Chapter Three) is of little surprise, as this became a set trope of Nazi antisemitic propaganda. It reached its nadir in Fritz Hippler's 1940 pseudo-documentary film *The Eternal Jew*, made by Goebbels's central party propaganda office, which opens with a map of Europe being overrun by rats bringing the Black Death to its inhabitants. The Nazi Party's monthly review of the film was subtitled 'The Film of a 2,000-year Rat Migration'.[39] On 20 January 1942, in a plush villa on the Wannsee in leafy suburban Berlin, the protocol outlining the plan for the murder of Europe's Jews was drafted. The Jews, it stated, were carriers of epidemics, and presented an extreme danger demanding a 'final solution'. Words have consequences.

What is fascinating about the rise of an analogous placing of blame in 2020 is that it was not the Jews but the Chinese who were said to be the 'foreigners' who brought the plague into the United States, even if, as it actually turned out, it initially arrived with returning wealthy vacationers and business people. When a ban on such travel was eventually instituted, Americans coming from even the worst-impacted areas of Europe were exempted. Indeed, one of Trump's claims to having mitigated the pandemic, one that he repeated over and over again as it was truly his only real talking point, was that he restricted travel from China in January 2020. The motivation for this was clear at the time: it had little to do with the spread of the virus, as it did not stop everyone from travelling to the United States from the PRC, only citizens of the PRC. China has functioned and continues to function for the United States, itself also an imagined community, as an eternal Other. There have been enough anti-Chinese voices, both left and right, to allow Trump to block citizens of the PRC but permit the return of Americans, defining them as part of the healthy American imagined community. At the time this was understood as part of his anti-Chinese trade offence.[40] (A year later it was the PRC that blocked foreigners and PRC citizens abroad from entering the country to back up its claim that the novel coronavirus was a threat from overseas.)

What one can observe, in parallel to the case of 1918 to 1933, is that the groups that coalesced around the sense of victimization did indeed foreground the economic imperative as one of their major claims. We can see that quite often it was those groups which had not benefited greatly from the gradual economic expansion following the 2008 'Great Recession' and Trump's bogus claim that his was the strongest American economy on record. It was clear, after the 2017 reduction of federal taxes primarily on the very wealthy, who received more than a 40 per cent reduction, that the elimination of many deductions that the working class as well as the middle class had relied on to shelter some of their income did not improve their economic lot. Rural groups, such as farmers, had actually seen major reversals in their economic stability because of Trump's tariff wars, and specific economic activities earmarked as targets for improvement during Trump's 2016 campaign, such as the coal industry, did substantially worse over the four years of his term. Yet the claim that his was the 'best economy ever' seems to have solidified his support.[41] Voting patterns in the 2020 presidential election reflected this as the Republicans held on to a number of state and local offices exactly because of the collective belief that the voters would be better off, over the long run, represented by self-labelled conservative economic policy. We can add to this that debt, long a bugaboo of the Republican Party, turned out not to be such a major problem during the four years of the Trump presidency. Suddenly in 2020 this became a major talking point in the election as well as in the halls of Congress, at least after the Joe Biden victory. All this played into establishing the victim status of those claiming that the pandemic was overinflated, used by malevolent forces, or indeed was the very creation of these forces.

Victims: Vaccines

Let us imagine how such constituent groups constituted themselves as victims and how the articulation of victimhood in one sphere begins to impact on the others. The notion that there had to be an objective correlative to the symbolic register employed has to be immediately abandoned, as the claims of each of these constituent groups are based on an ideological construct rather than lived experience. And this is true across all groups that labelled themselves as victims of the COVID-19 pandemic, as public health authorized and began to enforce, even in a limited way, the traditional means of combating viral infections. Employing means of social control that were used even well before germ theory, as we can see in Blackstone, became the core of pandemic responses after the late nineteenth century, even during the 1918 Spanish flu pandemic, during the first age of modern biology. What is vital to understand is that, as a commentator from McGill University's Office of Science and Society puts it, all these 'victim groups' 'have a commonality: protesting the COVID-19 lockdowns. Coverage from these protests often show people holding signs slapped with anti-vaccine rhetoric next to pro-militia activists and white supremacists.'[42] In other words, their symbolic registers have little or nothing to do with one another.

In early January 2017, immediately after taking office, Trump summoned Robert F. Kennedy Jr to Trump Tower to discuss his position on vaccination being the primary cause of autism, a position debunked with the withdrawal by the editors of *The Lancet* of a 1998 paper by British physician Andrew Wakefield in 2010. (Trump actually met with Wakefield, who had in the meantime relocated to Texas, in August 2016, encouraging the idea that he would be a welcome figure in the new administration.) Kennedy stated after his meeting with Trump that during the meeting he had accepted the offer of a position on the commission studying the relationship. Kennedy, the nephew of the murdered liberal president John F. Kennedy, commented that

> President-elect Trump has some doubts about the cur-
> rent vaccine policies, and he has questions about it . . .
> His opinion doesn't matter, but the science does matter,
> and we ought to be reading the science, and we ought to
> be debating the science. And that everybody ought to be
> able to be assured that the vaccines that we have – he's
> very pro-vaccine, as am I – [are] as safe as they possibly
> can be.[43]

While neither the commission nor Kennedy's appointment actually came to fruition, this associated Trump with a vocal leader of the cultural left. Kennedy was at the time clearly a leader of the global 'clean environment' movement. Speaking in Edmonton, Alberta (Canada), as the attorney for the Waterkeepers Alliance, an international organization that uses the courts to force industry and government to live up to environmental legislation, he advocated for rigid and strict national standards:

> One of the things they love to say in Ottawa and in Washington is, 'Let's get rid of the federal environmental laws and we'll return control to the provinces and the states.' After all, that's local control and it's community control and that's the essence of democracy . . . The real outcome of that devolution will not be local control. It will be corporate control, because these large corporations can so easily dominate the local political landscape.[44]

After his visit to Trump, Kennedy could have articulated a strong answer to Trump's four-year crusade to destroy *all* federal limits on environmental damage, across *all* the federal departments. But, of course, he did not. Rather he became the national anti-vaxxing spokesperson. Thus Kennedy and through him the environmental left became to a degree part of the symbolic world that inhabits the image of Donald Trump.

Trump had espoused anti-vaxxing views as early as 2007: 'When I was growing up, autism wasn't really a factor. And now all of a sudden, it's an epidemic . . . My theory, and I study it because I have young children, my theory is the shots. We're giving these massive injections at one time, and I really think it does something to the children.'[45] He repeated it again during a Republican presidential debate in September 2015: 'Just the other day, 2 years old, 2½ years old, a child, a beautiful child went to have the vaccine and came back, and a week later got a tremendous fever, got very, very sick, now is autistic.'[46] Yet one of the central claims about the success of the Trump presidency after the election is that

> he launched Operation Warp Speed, the greatest public health achievement in history. Until now, the record for the fastest vaccine development was four years. Operation Warp Speed did it in nine months. Because of Operation Warp Speed, the worst of the pandemic should be over by the spring. For all his mistakes in managing the pandemic, Trump is also responsible for ending it.[47]

Yet we need to note that Robert F. Kennedy Jr's response to the mRNA vaccines, on his organization's website, warned about the risks of the new vaccine, echoing his earlier objections to immunization in general.[48] He further argued that it was the pharmaceutical industry that was furthering its own interests in supporting this, ignoring the risks: 'We clearly have a systematic problem when government health regulators have utterly abdicated their responsibility to safeguard public health and refer safety concerns about shoddily tested, zero-liability vaccines to pharmaceutical companies.'[49] This 'anti-capitalist' argument is one from the American left, not the traditional American right.

Trump's own tweets and comments concerning vaccine development seemed to so politicize the issue that in September 2020 the nine major pharmaceutical companies involved publicly stated that the speed of their research and their desire for FDA approval had to be driven by the science, not by the political desires of the day. As the *Los Angeles Times* noted, 'Trump [was] vacillating: claiming credit for the delivery of the vaccines while trying to reassure those who are skeptical of the shots that he stands with them. On Sunday, Trump retweeted a video full of debunked conspiracy theories, including one that claimed the pandemic was manufactured as part of a plot to hurt him politically.'[50] But Robert F. Kennedy Jr was quite adamant in his anti-vaxxing argument, as his niece, Kerry Kennedy Meltzer, an internal medicine resident physician at New York-Presbyterian Hospital/Weill Cornell Medical Center, observed at the close of 2020 concerning the impact of such statements from her uncle and others:

> I recognize, with some trepidation, that people may wonder why I feel I need to speak out publicly about vaccines and against my uncle. The truth is, his name and platform mean that his views carry weight. After three hours, his Facebook post accusing government regulators of abdicating their responsibility to protect the public had 4,700 reactions, 2,300 shares and 641 comments. As a doctor, and as a member of the Kennedy family, I feel I must use whatever small platform I have to state a few things unequivocally. I love my uncle Bobby. I admire him for many reasons, chief among them his decades-long fight for a cleaner environment. But when it comes to vaccines, he is wrong.[51]

The initial response of the anti-vaxxers was that the risks outweighed the benefits. Yet Robert F. Kennedy Jr and the anti-vaxxers see themselves as an embattled minority struggling against a majoritarian society using bad science as a weapon. They are the victims, defending those at risk, not from the pandemic, but from the economic behemoth of the pharmaceutical industry and a compromised political system in its thrall. It is those opposed to vaccination who are the victims, as the right-wing TV commentator Glenn Beck observed:

> I'm interested in moving to common sense. I'm interested in moving in the direction of freedom . . . there's something happening . . . God gave me a brain. God gave me personal choice and responsibility for those choices, I'm going to say no to those vaccines because I've done my homework. Here's another group of people that are now being rounded-up and pointed at and called morons and idiots and crackpots and crazies. Just totally discredited . . . Where is anybody saying 'my gosh, we're living in the days of Galileo'? The church has become the state and if you don't practice their religion exactly the way they tell you to practice it, you're done.[52]

We know who the victims are and who the perpetrators are and the bright line between them cannot be overlooked. This is why, as we have observed above, the Holocaust quickly becomes the go-to model for such radical evil: for is there any evil worse in the public register of symbols than this?

The trajectory after the first vaccines were made widely available became evident over the next few months. 'Vaccine hesitancy' among many of the groups that it had been feared would avoid vaccination gave way to an increased demand for equity in access to the vaccines. As both were ramped up and the daily total of injections passed 2 million, there seemed to be an amelioration of the anxieties about the vaccines. Even Donald J. Trump and his wife received their vaccinations, indeed even before leaving the White House on 20 January, though in private and without any public announcement. Three of the other former presidents, George Bush, Bill Clinton and Barack Obama, had their vaccinations broadcast as public service announcements. Yet Trump as usual wished to play both sides of the argument: the pandemic is no big deal/the pandemic needs to be controlled. 'Everyone should go get your shot,' Trump said during his otherwise vindictive speech at Conservative Political Action Conference on 28 February.[53] In his first 'official' statement as a former president, published on 10 March 2021, he claimed, not incorrectly, credit for the rapid development of the vaccine on his watch. 'I hope everyone remembers when they're getting the COVID-19 (often referred to as the China Virus) Vaccine, that if I wasn't President, you wouldn't be getting that beautiful "shot" for 5 years, at best, and probably wouldn't be getting it at all.'[54] Yet Trump's previous anti-vaxxing views and his downplaying of the pandemic in the light of ever-increasing levels of morbidity and mortality had had a real-world impact on vaccine hesitation. While African Americans, ultra-Orthodox Jews and individuals from every corner of the economy and of every age, gender and ethnicity queued to get the vaccine, one group stood out and rejected it. According to a PBSNews-Hour/NPR/Marist poll taken the first week of March 2021, 49 per cent of men who self-identified as Republicans said they had no plans to get the vaccine.[55] That would, of course, include those African American, ultra-Orthodox or White nationalist followers of the former president. Words, we have said repeatedly in this book, have their consequences. Not history, not theology, not economics, but ideology had poisoned the public health well. By politicizing the public's health, Trump and his followers placed not only themselves but others at risk. Not freedom but licence rules in this symbolic domain, where taking credit for the vaccines and yet opposing their use is to be found, not cancelling each other out, but providing cover for the seeming resolution of the resulting double bind in favour of an anti-government stance.

Victims: Masks

Anti-maskers as well as those opposed to government-ordered lockdowns also made a claim to being the ultimate victims of oppression, basing this on poorly understood science, as did anti-vaxxers. Again, it is the abstract 'government' or an abstract 'science' that is the perpetrator. Trump marginalized masks on 3 April 2020 ('It's voluntary. You don't have to do it') but advocated them on 21 July ('I will use it gladly. And I say: If you can, use the mask'). Yet he did not model best practice health behaviours, rarely wearing a mask – and then only a dark blue one with a presidential seal – in public until 12 July 2020, when he visited Walter Reed National Military Hospital, after he had already begun large pre-election rallies, which became super-spreader events.[56] Symbols were in conflict, but as with vaccination, most of his followers 'knew' where he stood. One needs to note here that such events were often attended by symbolically unmasked political allies and acolytes, such as the 2016 Black presidential candidate Herman Cain, who died on 30 July 2020 after exposure to the virus, which most probably occurred at Trump's 20 June 2020 rally in Tulsa, Oklahoma. Cain had been vociferous in his public anti-masking advocacy, as he tweeted in June in regard to another Trump rally: 'Masks will not be mandatory for the event, which will be attended by President Trump. PEOPLE ARE FED UP!'[57]

The bully pulpit of the presidency was thus not incidentally contradictory in its messaging but provided every group over time with a set of images reinforcing their own positions, irrespective of ideology.[58] Trump knew that the masks were effective, just as he understood the virus's real and present danger at the very beginning of the pandemic, as Bob Woodward revealed in his account *Rage*, published in September 2020. His Secretary of Health and Human Services, Alex M. Azar II, briefed him on a Japanese study documenting the effectiveness of face masks, telling him: 'We have the proof. They work.' As a former senior advisor to the White House noted, 'making masks a culture war issue was the dumbest thing imaginable.' Yet Trump needed to appeal to all factions of the mask-wearing crowd while keeping clearly in mind that his anti-authoritarian, rather than libertarian, base 'will revolt,' as his chief-of-staff Mark Meadows noted.[59] And revolt they did.

In 2003, during the SARS pandemic in Hong Kong, mask wearing was an anti-authoritarian political statement, but in 2020, during the current pandemic in the United States, masks became a visible sign of victimization (and, one can add, of a lack of manliness and courage). Having been mocked publicly for having hidden in the White House bunker during the 'Black Lives Matter' demonstrations in Washington on 29 May 2020, and having staged his infamous walk across Lafayette Park on 1 June to show his manliness by waving a Bible at the cameras in the almost entirely complete absence of the demonstrators driven out by armed troops and police, Trump felt that he needed to prove this again during the first debate with Joe Biden at the beginning of October. Trump chose the mask as his symbol, mocking Biden as weak and feckless. 'I don't wear face masks like him. Every time you see him he's got a mask. He could be speaking 200 feet away . . . and he shows up with the biggest mask I've ever seen.'[60] The mask, perhaps read now as a sign of weakness, becomes for a number of communities on the right a symbol that transcends its public health function.

We can take one more case of community-forming symbols, this time on the political right. On 2 January 2016 an armed group of some forty far-right self-appointed vigilantes occupied a bird reserve, the Malheur National Wildlife Refuge in rural Oregon. Perhaps expecting park rangers engaged in birdwatching, they were soon under siege by federal marshals. During the occupation one of their members was killed confronting the federal officers and the rest were finally arrested on 11 February 2016. They were led by Ammon Bundy, who became a national spokesman for those opposed to the Bureau of Land Management and the federal supervision of lands in the West. He quickly became a folk hero to libertarians and anti-government ideologues. Bundy's position concerning governmental overreach was clear in these actions, and to no one's surprise he became one of the leaders in opposing the very low-key stay-at-home order issued by Republican governor Brad Little on 26 March 2020 in his home state of Idaho. Bundy stated that he would 'help provide legal, political and physical defense to people who are pressured by the "authorities" or anybody else to comply with the order'.[61]

After the state finally issued a mask mandate in August 2020, Bundy and other armed members of the so-called 'Patriot Movement' were arrested on 25 August while occupying (without masks, of course) the Idaho House of Representatives. When released, they returned the next day to occupy the chambers again, when he was again arrested. 'We don't believe they have a right to tell us that we have to put a manmade filter over our face to go outside,' Bundy said. 'It's not about, you know, the mandates or the mask. It's about them not having that right to do it.'[62] Keith Reynolds, the director of the Idaho Department of

Administration, following the views of the Idaho House Speaker Scott Bedke as well as the Senate President Pro Tempore Brent Hill, stated officially that 'Based on the totalitarian [*sic*] of the circumstances, I find that your refusal to comply with lawful orders of government officials and peace officers threatens to interfere with or impede the conduct of legitimate businesses and the primary uses of state facilities. You also present a threat to disrupt the legitimate business conducted here.'[63] Bundy was consistent, advocating against vaccination, or perhaps only against vaccination mandates, late in 2020 together with other groups such as 'Freedom Angels 2.0'. In April 2020 he was picketing the home of a policeman who had arrested an anti-vaxxer, Sarah Walton Brady, who was protesting at a closed playground.[64]

The idea that Bundy would contest state rules for public order in regard to the pandemic does not provoke much surprise, any more than Robert Kennedy Jr's use of this platform to advocate for his own anti-vaxxer position. But like Kennedy's, Bundy's anti-governmental stance during the pandemic was complex. In late May 2020, well into the pandemic, after the homicide of George Floyd in Minneapolis, Minnesota, Bundy openly supported the widespread demonstrations. In a video he stated that he was going to attend 'a rally with the Black Lives Matter in support of defunding the police because yes the police need to be defunded'. He was deterred by the fear that his right-wing associates in the 'Patriot Movement' would physically attack him. 'You must have a problem in your mind if you think that somehow the Black Lives Matter is more dangerous than the police,' he said. 'You must have a problem in your mind if you think that Antifa is the one going to take your freedom.'[65] (Antifa is the collective name for those loosely organized activists opposed to right-wing fascism.) Here we can fast forward to 6 January

2021 and the insurrection at the Capitol. There, American flags defaced with a blue stripe to signify right-wing support of the police and the 'Blue Lives Matter' movement were used to beat the police defending the Capitol. When conservative commentators observed this that day (and then subsequently during Congressional hearings), the answer was that it could not have been Trump supporters but rather 'Antifa or BLM or other insurgents' in disguise.[66] The conflict within their symbolic worldview was resolved and they knew who had to be at fault.

Here Lockean 'freedom' becomes the touchstone for the privilege now attended to all who are affiliated in their opposition to any and all public health interventions. Without seeming flip, one does want to quote the popular example given by the legal philosopher Zechariah Chafee Jr in the June 1919 issue of the *Harvard Law Review*: 'Each side takes the position of the man who was arrested for swinging his arms and hitting another in the nose, and asked the judge if he did not have a right to swing his arms in a free country. "Your right to swing your arms ends just where the other man's nose begins."'[67] This statement is seemingly apposite for the age of COVID-19, paraphrased perhaps as 'just where the other man's mask begins'.

Freedom to Infect

Freedom seems to be an infinitely expandable category across all fields of endeavour, as the ultra-conservative Catholic Supreme Court Justice Samuel Alito observed in a speech to the Federalist Society in which he declared that 'religious liberty is fast becoming a disfavored right' because of public health restrictions. He, like Trump, argued both sides of the issue simultaneously, claiming not to be 'diminishing the virus' threat to public health' or questioning the 'legality of COVID restrictions'. But he noted, 'We have never before seen restrictions as severe, extensive and prolonged as those experienced for most of 2020.' (Evidently he was ignorant of the massive social controls introduced, admittedly just as unsystematically, across the various states in 1918.) The courts (including later the Supreme Court) split in 2020 on the issue of which right was the primary one, the right to protect life or the unfettered right to public worship. He commented in his speech on a Nevada case upholding occupancy limitations in places of public gathering: 'Take a quick look at the Constitution. You will see the free-exercise clause of the First Amendment, which protects religious liberty. You will not find a craps clause, or a blackjack clause, or a slot machine clause.'[68] Joining the majority opinion during the successful court case, mentioned in Chapter Three, brought by Agudath Israel and the Diocese of Brooklyn against measures in New York State on 25 November 2020, such a public health limitation

> violates the free exercise clause as targeting and a religious gerrymander when [Governor Andrew] Cuomo made clear through unambiguous statements that the order was targeted at a religious minority's practices and traditions; and (2) whether the provisions of that order limiting in-person 'house of worship' attendance to 10 or 25 people, while allowing numerous secular businesses to operate without any capacity restrictions, violate the free exercise clause on its face by disfavoring worship.[69]

Alito in this case simply supported the conversative majority, radically shifting the court's earlier position in May 2020 in *South Bay United Pentecostal Church v. Newsom* (140 S. Ct. 1613, 2020), in a narrow 5-4 decision (Justice Ruth Bader Ginsburg was still alive): public health precautions were the right not only of governmental entities but of individuals. In this earlier finding the court had held that there was a 'compelling government interest', the litmus test for such cases under the First Amendment, in controlling the pandemic: in other words, keep your fist away from our mask-covered noses.

By the end of 2020 Hobbes's 'public sword' seemed to have been weakened if not abandoned by the U.S. Supreme Court, which placed 'freedom of religion' above the public's health. However, the massive spikes in morbidity and mortality beginning in December 2020 led the court, meeting virtually because of the pandemic, to revisit the question of state imposition of public health rules on religious practice in the case of *South Bay United Pentecostal Church v. Newsom*. The new conservative majority held again that a state must be more limited in the strictures imposed on a house of worship than on other institutions, giving at least lip service to the clear fact that their determination did not follow 'the science'. Justice Neil M. Gorsuch, writing for himself and two others in the majority, wrote, 'Of course we are not scientists, but neither may we abandon the field when government officials with experts in tow seek to infringe a constitutionally protected liberty.'[70] (We can note that this is the caveat employed by right-wing climate-science deniers to dismiss the scientific consensus about the radical climate emergency at the same moment. 'I am not a scientist . . .'.[71]) He concluded with the claim, refuted already in the first footnote to the majority decision, that 'If Hollywood may host a studio audience or film a singing competition while not a single soul may enter California's churches, synagogues, and mosques, something has gone seriously awry.' Writing for the minority, Justice

Elena Kagan laid out the case against lifting the limitations most clearly:

> Justices of this Court are not scientists. Nor do we know much about public health policy. Yet today the Court displaces the judgments of experts about how to respond to a raging pandemic. The Court orders California to weaken its restrictions on public gatherings by making a special exception for worship services. The majority does so even though the State's policies treat worship just as favorably as secular activities (including political assemblies) that, according to medical evidence, pose the same risk of COVID transmission. Under the Court's injunction, the State must instead treat worship services like secular activities that pose a much lesser danger.

The majority's opinion would seem to be consistent with the earlier finding. But Hobbes's demand for some protection of the body politic has now been acknowledged. Although in the first instance the court marginalized science, it moderated its stance by following the very same scientific principle (or advice) here, for it held here that there was a 'compelling government interest', the litmus test for such cases under the First Amendment, in controlling the pandemic: in other words, keep your fist away from our mask-covered nose. Yet by the beginning of April 2021, they stopped the State of California from limiting attendance at religious services held in private homes (*Ritesh Tandon, et al. v. Newsom*), while admonishing the California courts for ignoring the Supreme Court's inconsistent findings stating that religious practice is more important than the public's health. The 5 to 4 decision stressed the primacy of religious freedom, even though the court's minority pointed out that the faulty analogy of the majority that such religious services were equivalent to retail stores and hair salons ignored the actual length of and activities during such religious services and the evident fact that such services had spread the virus to their participants in other cases. So maybe religious establishments really are potential super-spreader sites and one's freedom of religion is not harmed by society claiming that they actually exacerbate the spread of the pandemic. 'Not being scientists', here the justices in the majority actually were swayed by science. The health of the collective can be more important even than religious freedom in such contexts. Courts can learn that the codes concerning health risk and ideology, which clearly compete in 2021, sometimes need to have their symbolic registers merged, even when they are clearly antithetical.

Everyone has a voice in this world of COVID-19, except of course the more than half a million dead in the United States at the violent conclusion of Trump's term in office, whose individual rights ended at their interments. Since such lumping together of 'freedoms' is now part of a global response to all interventions to ameliorate the pandemic, from France to the UK, from Australia to Germany, the alliances that have been formed merge and confuse all the symbolic registers originally defining each community. This anxiety is fuelled by a long-standing response to germ theory that denies the efficacy of allopathic medicine; indeed, labels it as poisonous and destructive to health and welfare. The Nazis fuelled this when 'Reichsärzteführer' Gerhard Wagner argued in 1933 that *Naturheilkunde* (alternative and complementary) medicine must take its place parallel to clinical (allotropic) medicine. In 1935 he was instrumental in founding the *Arbeitsgemeinschaft für eine Neue Deutsche Heilkunde*

(Working Group for a New German Alternative Medicine), and then attempted to merge this organization with the official state medical society. That did not happen because of the opposition of medically trained physicians, who feared losing status. By 1937 he ended his attempt to merge both, but alternative medicine remained within modern German healthcare, even when homeopathic physicians came to have medical degrees. This was a little different in the United States: Andrew Still's 'osteopathy', developed in the early 1890s as an alternative therapy, became a sub-set of allopathic medicine, unlike chiropractic, by the close of the century, ensuring its practitioners equal status to allopathic physicians. These tensions increased in the twenty-first century, often endorsed by celebrities and multiplied on social media. As with big pharmaceuticals, 'natural' herbal medicines are big business too. It is of little surprise that COVID-19 cures appeared simultaneously in both spheres of medical practice. Thus in the world of alternative and complementary medicine, labelled 'folk medicine' in Germany and 'traditional medicine' by the WHO, there was the claim that ginger root and meteorite dust could 'cure' the virus.[72] But quackery was not limited to this arena. Some had an allopathic imprimatur, such as the advocates of hydroxychloroquine as a treatment for the virus. This was advocated on the public stage by Donald Trump in July 2020 and then obsessively seconded by the economist Peter Navarro, Trump's policy coordinator on employing the Defense Production Act to produce PPE, ventilators and other materials for use against the pandemic. Even more importantly, after August 2020, it was advocated by the Stanford University-based neuroradiologist Scott Atlas, whose anti-masking stance endeared him to Donald Trump and moved Trump to appoint him to the Coronavirus Task Force in August 2020. Quackery promises 'magic bullets' that do not disturb the symbolic world that the believers inhabit, no matter how abstruse or contradictory.

Throw in to this mix of pandemic worldviews the now global QAnon conspiracy that makes Donald Trump a divine intercessor in a process of overcoming deep-seated corruption signalled by paedophilia and child murder (think of the historic blood libels across the globe), and brings back to a shadow life Robert F. Kennedy Jr's cousin John F. Kennedy Jr as one of its 'white knights', and one can see how both complex and simple such systems have become.[73] All can add to them their own vocabulary of symbols defining their own communities and see in all the others not merely allies but, even stranger, mirror images of themselves. They are all victims: of the 'Nazis' in power today, of the secret cabals just visible ever so slightly under the surface, of a state run amok to control what is in essence a hoax perpetrated by elites, the banks, the media, the 5G networks, or all of the above. Our focus here has been on the United States, but the core problem exists across a wide range of nation-states, from the Netherlands to Sweden to Brazil, indeed, to Germany. All the rioting mobs have taken their rhetoric, and their slogans (often in English), from the American model. Globalism, so often decried as one of the causes of the Right's discomfort, comes to be part of the Right's creation of itself as a global community.

The Absolute Rights of Man

Conservatives used to make a working distinction between freedom and licence. And as we began with William Blackstone's *Commentaries on the Laws of England*, defining our obligations in times of plague, let us conclude here with the opening lines of his classic work in which he pits the importance of freedom against our obligations to the greater good that defines what law and society are:

> THE absolute rights of man, considered as a free agent, endowed with discernment to known good from evil, and with power of choosing those measures which appear to him to be most desirable, are usually summed up on one general appellation, and denominated the natural liberty of mankind. This natural liberty consists properly in a power of acting as one thinks fit, without any restraint or control, unless by the law of nature . . . But every man, when he enters into society, gives up a part of his natural liberty, as the price of so valuable a purchase; and, in consideration of receiving the advantages of mutual commerce, obliges himself to conform to those laws, which the community has thought proper to establish . . . Hence, we may collect that the law, which restrains a man from doing mischief to his fellow citizens, though it diminishes the natural, increases the civil liberty of mankind.[74]

'Facultas ejus, quod cuique facere libet, nisi quid jure prohibetur' – all is allowed but that which is prohibited by law. But hidden within Blackwell's claim to the primacy of the law is the Hippocratic prohibition in the *Epidemics*, 'primum non nocere', first do no harm. Here too we can see how black letter law demands our acknowledgement of the limitations of our embeddedness in a social fabric that may well transcend the symbolic regime through which we define our imagined community.

The Enlightenment, at least Immanuel Kant, added to this the not unimportant nuance that the laws must have been acceded to by the people over which they will have domination. For Kant duty to others is central to all moral law, rather than crass self-interest or even self-preservation. And COVID-19 has shown how very easy even the best and most comprehensive public health regimes can be exploited, as in Hungary, Serbia and the Philippines, for less than democratic aims.[75] Yet Kant is clear: 'I ought never to act except in such a way that I could also will that my maxim should become a universal law.'[76] This is nothing new or even surprising. As the cornerstone of Blackstone's logic, underlying all British Common Law seems to be a basic moral assumption encompassing the teaching of Jesus in the Sermon on the Mount: 'All things whatsoever ye would that men should do to you, do ye even so to them' (Matthew 7:12) or Rabbi Hillel's answer to the man who ironically asks him whether he can teach him all Jewish law standing on one foot: 'That which is despicable to you, do not do to your fellow, this is the whole Torah, and the rest is commentary, go and learn it' (Babylonian Talmud: Shabbat 31a).

Four centuries before Hillel, living in the midst of great turmoil, Confucius and his students (known as the early Confucians) all revered ethical and moral teachers whose works echoed down the centuries, and taught that individual rights are embedded in social relations and subject to the obligations associated with those relationships. This was done to help people coping with change and loss and to bring cohesiveness to a society torn by continuous wars. They argued that one should place the self at the centre of relationships rather than simply exist as an isolated individual. Society is a community of trust rather than merely a system of adversarial relationships; human beings are duty-bound to respect their family, society and state: 'To establish oneself is to help others to establish themselves; To enlarge oneself is to help others to enlarge themselves' (*Analects* 6: 28).

We can add one further interpretation to this notion of the individual's debt to the collective. In his *Civilization and Its Discontents* (1930) Sigmund Freud reads the 'Golden Rule' that haunts religion as an extension precisely of those taboos that structure the superego. For Freud all ethical considerations are part of the function of the superego, impressed upon the individual so that society can 'get rid of the greatest hindrance to civilization – namely, the constitutional inclination of human beings to be aggressive towards one another'. Ethics seem logical, indeed rational, but at the end they are merely made concrete in 'the most recent of the cultural commands of the super-ego, the commandment to love one's neighbour as oneself'.[77] Perhaps at the end of the day, in regard to COVID-19, Freud is right. We have seen the veneer of civilization easily peeled back as we have been confronted with what we believe to be our risk from overwhelming forces, invisible, implacable, such as the virus. This has undermined all those collective reassurances we normally have to balance our sense of instability. We now seek for meaning where little meaning can actually exist; and we fall back on those symbolic realms that provide us, often falsely, with that assurance. Trump was the concretization of that assurance, and the deaths on his watch proof of its falsity.

What has evolved over the course of the COVID-19 pandemic among some groups, now more or less equally labelled oppositional, is the abandonment of community and the assertion of a false claim to autonomy of choice. This is defined in terms of the imagined community where all such are allied in their claims for individual autonomy. The contradictions work themselves out in practice and in the deaths of those not even peripherally involved in their world. As in Milton Rokeach's 1964 *Three Christs of Ypsilanti*, the account of three paranoid schizophrenics sitting in the asylum claiming to be the Saviour preaching at the Mount of Olives, each is able to negotiate a space that works for them in the totality of the symbolic regimes encompassing often contradictory notions of autonomy.

6

MARGINALITY AND DISEASE

In 1988 Charles E. Rosenberg, the doyen of American medical historians, wrote an essay on AIDS which began,

> AIDS has reminded us of some very old truths, truths most Americans had managed to forget during the past decades. Epidemic infectious disease is not simply a historical phenomenon – or one limited like famine to the non-white remote continents. By the end of the 1970s, most Americans had come to regard themselves as no longer at risk; infectious disease was almost by definition amenable to medical intervention. Not since the last severe polio threats more than a quarter century ago has the United States experienced the collective fear of epidemic disease.

The footnote to this paragraph, a paragraph seemingly as valid today as in 1988, read: 'Influenza does not seem to have the same ability to inspire widespread fear – in part because we have also forgotten the 1918 flu epidemic.'[1] Forgetting collective fear is a common phenomenon after a crisis. Whether a pandemic ends in a bang or a whimper, it is always followed by amnesia. We have classic repression documented even on the part of Holocaust survivors and survivors of the Great Leap Forward famine in the PRC, but the reality is that such 'forgetting' is never forgotten.[2] Individuals repress; individuals in collectives use those symbols that define their community to deal with collective fear. Like viruses, these symbols are just bits of information; they are always present, but remain inert. It is the cells in our body and brain that bring them to life. There is also the tendency of yearning for 'normality', which leads society to forget the cracks that need fixing. Our responses to pandemic are always social, even though the symbolic register of the pandemic is medicalized. David Rieff, in his extraordinary study of the necessary fragility of historical memory, quotes La Rochefoucauld: 'No man can stare for long at death or the sun.'[3] Remembering has its own pitfalls, and while it may be a moral duty (pace Paul Ricoeur), it is never a pleasant one. Friedrich Nietzsche, in 'The Use and Abuse of History' (1872), argued that remembering is being able selectively to forget the totality of the past and thus shape it into a system useful for what he calls 'life', our quotidian existence. Thus if a collective seems to remember, it is only through the fragmented, inchoate symbolic registers cobbled together in the very act of remembering which continually shape individual memory. Our pandemic past is never dead; indeed, it is truly never past, to paraphrase William Faulkner, imagining the legacy of the Civil War in mid-twentieth-century America.

Rosenberg's evocation in 1988 of the Spanish flu having been repressed rather than sublimated into the texts that followed the First World War is telling, for over the past decade there have been massive attempts to reveal how writers and painters evoked exactly this sublimated experience well into the post-Second World War era.[4] W. B. Yeats and T. S. Eliot, both infected or living with infected spouses, incorporated their experiences into 'The Second Coming' and *The Waste Land*, poems that echo throughout the twentieth century, along with the fiction of Katherine Anne Porter, Virginia Woolf and Ernest Hemingway. Yet these texts were always mediated by the aesthetics shaping their representation and reception, which is why we need to work very hard to excavate the pandemic's presence. Spiritualism, so rampant after the First World War, desired to reach out to those killed in the war in a direct and unmediated manner; recall Arthur Conan Doyle's obsession with Spiritualism in order to reach his late son Kingsley, dead at the Somme, or Oliver J. Lodge's best-selling account of memory and love that transcend death in his *Raymond; or, Life and Death* (1916), named after his son, dead at Ypres. No such attempts are made to reach the influenza dead. But Elizabeth Outka reminds us of the post-pandemic absence of the 1918 influenza and its intense presence brilliantly when she concludes her study with the observation that

> A lethal pandemic leaves few tangible reminders behind. No buildings collapse. No battlefields or crash sites are preserved. Rarely do memorials mark its passing. Its effects are felt everywhere but located in no particular place, except perhaps in the bodies and memories of the living who remain . . . The pandemic produced so many layers of loss – the loss of life, the loss those deaths produced for loved ones, the loss of health for many survivors, and the loss of the event itself in so many of our histories. We can account for the impact of the pandemic, but how do we represent the loss?[5]

What she warns us of is that 'even a modern catastrophic pandemic *that has already happened* can be hidden, unless we learn to read for its presence.'[6] This book, written in the midst of a global pandemic, is an attempt to read its impact on collectives, on communities, rather than on individuals, be they writers and artists or simply those who experienced it in their daily lives. It is an attempt to examine the 'few tangible reminders' as they are presented to us over the course of the pandemic. Forgetting, repression or, as some have now called it, 'corona fatigue' seems at the moment possible only if one targets others to assuage one's anxieties and fears.

The act of repression, or 'cognitive inertia', as one historian observes, means that each and every recurrence of such an event, even tangentially, reinscribes the anxiety and the need to seek a source to blame. Since in 1918 'many of those in the uninfected areas underestimated the danger posed by the Spanish flu because cognitive inertia – the tendency of existing beliefs or habits of thought to blind people to changed realities . . . The effects of cognitive inertia are by definition unrecognized by those who experience it.'[7] Unrecognized or repressed? For in 1918 there were certainly sufficient people who were old enough to have experienced epidemics of malaria (which regularly appeared in the West until the late 1940s), yellow fever (massively present in 1905), cholera (last in 1910–11, part of a global pandemic) and even bubonic plague (the Black Death, regularly reappearing in the West until the 1920s). Never mind annual and intense epidemics of polio, measles and other infectious diseases that were endemic to the West.[8] The irony in 2020 in the West is that it was not the working through of the pandemics of the age of our grandparents and parents but the Black Death, that curse earlier blamed on the Jews, that reappeared over and over again. William Shakespeare was quarantined during the various epidemics of plague from 1582 to 1603 and beyond, during which it has been variously claimed that his brother or his son perished, and that he as a result wrote *King Lear*, in which Lear curses Goneril as 'A plague-sore, or embossed carbuncle / In my corrupted blood' (2: 4). Claims that, as with the literary figures telling their tales in Boccaccio's *Decameron* (1353), plague, quarantine and the constant fear of death lead to creativity, seem to have engaged those in lockdown for COVID-19, yet none of these claims are actually valid.[9] Plague kills; it demeans; it rarely uplifts, except in fiction. We yearn for the notion that our suffering, our losses, our 'lockdown fatigue' will be given meaning. We seek reassurance of the meaning our present lives must have in the distant past among works that we believe have stood the test of time. More than the maximum 10,000 citations for 'Shakespeare' and 'plague' appeared on Nexis after 1 March 2020.[10]

Epidemic/Pandemic

In all cases we need to remember in this age of forgetting that a pandemic or an epidemic is not a measure only of how widespread a disease actually is, but of how it is perceived. Epidemic (and its kissing cousin pandemic) may be a technical term from epidemiology for any 'large-scale temporary increase in the occurrence of a disease in a community or region, which is clearly in excess of normal expectancy, whereas a pandemic is the occurrence of a disease which is clearly in excess of normal expectancy and is spread over a whole geographical area, usually crossing national boundaries', as Daniel Reid notes in *The Oxford Companion to the Body*. Yet 'epidemic' maintains a powerful metaphorical connection to universal, lethal contagion from its earliest to its most recent use, because, as Reid begins his entry, 'the word "epidemic" has an emotional ring to it', which is 'why it is often used wrongly'.[11] 'Epidemic' as well as 'pandemic' have a strong metaphorical use in terms of the unfettered spread of deadly and uncontrolled diseases and the use of these terms has always had social and emotional consequences.

'Epidemic' seems to be a creation of the age of Shakespeare, borrowed from the French. Thomas Lodge in his 1603 *A Treatise of the Plague* needed to define this new notion for his readership: 'An Epidemick plague, is a common and popular sicknesse, happning in some region, or country, at a certaine time, caused by a certaine indisposition of the aire, or waters of the same region, producing in all sorts of people, one and the same sicknesse.'[12] By 1666 Gideon Harvey had added 'pandemic' to our vocabulary in his book on rickets, the 'English disease', *Morbus Anglicus*, noting the fear attendant to

Pandemick, or Endemick, or rather a Vernacular Disease
(a disease always reigning in a Countrey) . . . that is
a common disease owing its rise to some common
external and perennal (lasting all the year) cause of a
Countrey . . . And beyond this denomination the disease
may not improperly be stiled Epidemick (popular,) that
is, surprizing many at a certain season of the year . . .
it may be connumerated (numbred) with the worst of
Epidemicks (popular diseases,) since next to the Plague,
Pox, and Leprosy, it yeilds to none in point of Contagion
(catching).[13]

What is vital to our experience of covid-19 is that such terms quickly took on metaphorical and catastrophic meaning, as in John Milton's condemnation of the dissolution of bounds of faith in the second edition in 1644 of his treatise *Doctrine and Discipline of Divorce*: 'public dispensations of lewd uncleanness, the first good consequence of such a relax will be the justifying of papal stews, joined with a toleration of epidemic whoredom. Justice must revolt from the end of her authority, and become the patron of that whereof she was created the punisher.'[14] (Shakespeare had used neither 'epidemic' nor 'pandemic', but 'plague' was a constant metaphor that haunts most of his works, with 105 uses.) That ambiguity that links scientific description to metaphor continues in the age of COVID-19.

If HIV/AIDS created a mass panic as part of, not as a result of, the idea of an epidemic in the 1980s, it built on the repressed sense of fear inherent in the communities that had not only experienced polio but retained the repressed echoes of the Spanish flu.[15] Thus public health officials tended to be overly careful about evoking the past by speaking about global or even regional pandemics. On 21 May 2009 the World Health Organization's director-general, Margaret Chan, decided that influenza A (H1N1) was not going to become a pandemic. She had been the Director of Health in Hong Kong in 1997 and achieved visibility in combating the first human outbreak of H5N1 avian influenza before leading the fight against SARS in 2003. Her presence as a political as well as a public health figure during these pandemics led to her appointment as the director-general of the WHO in 2006. She understood the political implications of the term 'pandemic', not stemming from any epidemiological rationale but from the fact that the use of the term itself was feared to trigger global panic. 'Swine flu' would have become a stage six pandemic on that date. But Chan observed that 'I know that you have given me a lot of trust and flexibility, and this is not an easy task. I need to balance how science should play a role and not to forget about the people.'[16] Not 'science' but the public response was the key to the rethinking of what the outbreak of H1N1 should be labelled. By 11 June 2009 H1N1 was a designated pandemic.

This too had its political dimension with medical consequences. This is, of course, exactly parallel to the discussions within the WHO after the 4 January 2020 announcement of a 'cluster of pneumonia cases in Wuhan' concerning COVID-19. It was only on 11 March 2020 that the WHO labelled COVID-19 a 'pandemic'. Dr Tedros Adhanom Ghebreyesus, the director-general, stated that:

> Pandemic is not a word to use lightly or carelessly. It is a word that, if misused, can cause unreasonable fear, or unjustified acceptance that the fight is over, leading to unnecessary suffering and death. Describing the situation as a pandemic does not change WHO's assessment of the threat posed by this virus. It doesn't change what WHO is doing, and it doesn't change what countries should do. We have never before seen a pandemic sparked by a coronavirus. This is the first pandemic caused by a coronavirus.[17]

Words matter: terms charged with heavy metaphoric meaning change the way we see, imagine and fear infectious diseases.

With H1N1 Margaret Chan's comments were revealing, as they echo the effect that public health pronouncements have on the global public. It is easier to generate panic than it is to disseminate real information. And we had been there before, and not only in 1918. Richard Neustadt and Ernest May spelled out the dangers of epidemics when they looked at the 1976 swine flu debacle.[18] Swine flu was then seen as an imminent danger. The science of the time seemed to bear this out, as the virus's antigenic characteristics linked it to the 1918 influenza epidemic, at least in terms of the science of the day. In 1976 the 1918 Spanish flu seemed, as today, to be barely remembered, when it was invoked at all. Its evocation made moral panic about swine flu possible. Yet it was clear that it was the immediate evocation of the influenza epidemic of 1968, hardly on the same scale as 1918, that actually motivated the civil servants to act. Public health officials were revealed to have been woefully unprepared for that epidemic, which was seen as a political disaster given their claims of being in charge of the nation's public health. 'Beat '68' was the mantra in 1976; the 1918 influenza epidemic was the historical rationale. Remember that military historians say: 'We always fight the last war.' And that was 1968.

In 1976 the then head of the Center (later Centers) for Disease Control (CDC), David Sencer, needed to be seen as being prepared, in contrast to the panic that had attended the outbreak in 1968. As he noted, 'the Administration can tolerate unnecessary health expenditures better than unnecessary death and illness, particularly if a flu pandemic should occur.'[19] Money was no object when confronted with the very possibility of 1968 again. The power of Sencer's argument rested on the inescapable fact that there had been a recent unrelated outbreak of Legionnaires' disease in the mid-1970s. This 'epidemic' reinforced the public's acceptance that there might be the potential for an epidemic of 1918 proportions.

The public health claim was that all that was known about influenza pointed to quick action through vaccination as the most certain way to head off the epidemic. The CDC then used the horrors of 1918 as their 'worst-case scenario'. They saw safe, easily manufactured vaccines as the only escape. The power of the American presidency was harnessed to this claim and Gerald Ford became a major figure in disseminating the mass awareness of influenza, being vaccinated publicly in October 1976. The reality turned out quite differently in both cases. The swine flu vaccine in 1976 caused more harm in the normal morbidity associated with vaccination than the disease did itself. Indeed, Donald Trump raised this spectre in his debates with Joe Biden in advance of the November 2020 presidential election.[20] Avian influenza in the twenty-first century triggered international responses greatly out of scale to the actual danger.

These epidemics never materialized then, but these experiences did shape the official responses to COVID-19. This continued into the twenty-first century; as we discussed earlier, George W. Bush announced in 2005, having read John Barry's history of the 1918 pandemic, that a pandemic was potentially the world's greatest risk – replacing international terrorism, for a time. In 2020 all the false starts suddenly looked like well-thought-through rehearsals for Armageddon, but Donald Trump had abrogated all the earlier plans and fired all the team assembled by his predecessors. Trump not only undermined the scientists at the National Institutes of Health and the Food and Drug Administration but politicized the public health authorities in the CDC. Not only was the country ill prepared in 2020 but those institutions that should have been prepared turned to supporting Trump's political fantasies by subsuming their expertise to his political interest. Public health is political, that is true, but it needs to rest on the presuppositions of the science as undergirding policy rather than, as in 2020, narcissistic policy redefining the science and cherry-picking the data. This too has happened before in undermining the public's health, recently in the case of Thabo Mbeki's denialism and quack cures for HIV/AIDS that led to the death of 330,000 people in South Africa from 1999 to 2008. The question remains not why such a misdirection was undertaken but why the scientific spokespeople, with few notable exceptions such as Dr Francis Collins and Dr Anthony Fauci at NIH, were willing to be so manipulated. The end result was the complete disregard for expertise that continued well into 2021 on the part of Trump's supporters. Their moral panic became evident at the Capitol on 6 January, when the pandemic deniers, the anti-maskers, the Trump stalwarts, the conspiracy theorists, the anti-vaxxers, the antisemites and racists suddenly felt the floor falling away under their feet – a sensation that most Americans had experienced after the March 2020 lockdown.

Moral Panics

Some diseases cause moral panic, much as did syphilis in the nineteenth century and HIV/AIDS in the 1980s, with real political and social implications. We were in Hong Kong in December 2009. We saw the result of the re-emergence of moral panic present in that city reminiscent of the 2003 outbreak of another coronavirus pandemic, severe acute respiratory syndrome (SARS). It was the result of the moral opprobrium levelled at southern China as being the source of an illness that threatened the world. In 2009 everyone was hyper-aware of H1N1 influenza, from the city health officials who met you at the Hong Kong airport wearing masks and brandishing thermometers to the city's inhabitants, hidden behind their masks on the trams. When it first arose in southern China in 2003, SARS was dubbed 'severe acute nervousness syndrome' (*feidianxing shengjing bing*) because it was accompanied by almost paranoid fear.[21] Here the model of an infection as having a psychological component – public hysteria about vulnerability – was manifest.[22] The new disease was seen with much the same anxiety and paranoia in the West as a new cholera or Black Death spreading from the East along travel and economic routes would have been.

The experience of infectious disease can also have a powerful psychological impact. SARS quickly became a moral panic which spread worldwide, being accompanied by a true sense of stigma.[23] In the twenty-first century, spreading quickly by plane, rather than slowly by caravan as with the Black Death in the Middle Ages or by troop train during the Great Influenza in the early twentieth century, SARS was apocalyptically set to invade and destroy 'civilization'. The initial response in China was panic, as one of the authors of this book wrote at the time:

> Anti-SARS has now become a political movement in China. All officials are living in nightmares of being sacked. The police force are enforcing anti-SARS measures. Curfews have been introduced; people have been arrested for any minor illnesses. SARS is not only headlines; it has become the only topic of conversation. Ordinary people are living in great fear . . . though thousands of people are dying each day in China as a result of building accidents, no one seems to care and one hardly reads about them in the paper. Three thousand school children were poisoned by soy milk, but they were not allowed to be treated outside of the local hospital, so that the news would not spread. However, the hospital was poorly equipped to cope with the situation.[24]

Thereafter the general response was equally chaotic:

> After the national Minister of Health and the Mayor of Beijing were fired for 'covering up' the extent of the SARS epidemic, a historian in Beijing wrote me that 'Sacking two people is just another way of covering things up and

continuing to tell lies. It happens all the time in China, I am so used to it. Though I don't think I should get used to it. Sometimes I really feel I should say something . . . or perhaps not. Beijing is in total panic right now; people have lost their faith in the official report and the government. Everyone knows they are telling the lies, people don't know what to believe anymore. As a result, they turn to everyone and rush into drug stores to buy every imaginable medicine. They won't get killed by SARS but they are going to drug themselves to death! It's really quite awful.'[25]

And, according to public health authorities, like COVID-19, as discussed in Chapter Two, all this chaos began in the food chain.

Real infectious diseases do have a powerful psychological effect. SARS, like COVID-19, quickly became a moral panic which spread worldwide, accompanied by a true sense of stigma. Moral panics can alter the meaning and impact of real situations in the world. The term had its origin in Jock Young's study of the beginnings of the British drug scene. It has since been used to analyse 'social epidemics' and even 'pandemics' such as child abuse and, of course, the American 'war on drugs'.[26] No one would be fool-hardy enough to claim that child abuse or drug addiction does not exist, then or now, but the moral panic associated with these categories over the past decades is the result of heightened anxiety about social instability and the concomitant need to blame those seen as at fault for it. Obesity clearly exists in the world; but how it is defined is culturally, not scientifically, limited and its centrality in the mental universe of any given individual is heavily dependent on the role of anxiety associated with it. And yet we hear public health authorities across the world speak glibly of 'globesity', an global epidemic of obesity.

As the twentieth century ended, haunted by the millions of deaths from HIV/AIDS, still very much present globally in 2020 though less anxiety-producing since it has seemingly been mitigated through new therapies, a new millennium saw new pandemics, from SARS to swine flu and Ebola. Governments and people acted with the same sort of denial coupled with panic, but none reached the scale we see now with COVID-19. The wider context (with the global political transformation often combined with economic instability) of 2019 led to the public health/political disaster of 2020. This allowed people to externalize what had been repressed in each case, forgotten yet not forgotten. In 2020 the fear spread quickly by social media rather than slowly by newspapers and TV: COVID-19, it was claimed, was set to invade and destroy 'civilization'. And the residents of Wuhan, and then Orthodox Jews, and then people of colour, were targeted for this, each in their own way. For dominant aspects of White society,

> the mask has become the symbol of this moral panic, where wearing or not wearing one has come to reflect a repertoire of gendered forms of social distancing, from performances of male machismo through guns and defiance, to those of female helpfulness, care and compliance. Whether economic, medical, family-related, or social, the pandemic has made these issues, attitudes, and anxieties surface in stark ways.[27]

COVID-19, and earlier coronavirus epidemics, were serious health events, but our medical responses to them were determined as much by the social meaning associated with the diseases as the gradual development of medical knowledge and technology.

Constructing diseases does not always mean inventing them. Often, real pathological experiences are rethought as part of a new pattern that can then be discerned, diagnosed and treated. Our sense of our own risk and our response to that risk shape how we experience the illness itself. Thus H1N1 seems not to have had a very different presentation from that of seasonal influenza and, sadly, had about the same morbidity and mortality rates as that annual pandemic. But we were schooled by SARS and subsequently by the fear of avian influenza. Following the model of SARS, avian influenza became a focus of anxiety about epidemics. Although there was no avian influenza epidemic in 2004, 2005 or 2006, the WHO continued to map the spread of such a potential epidemic spread by wild birds crossing the wide Siberian distances and encroaching on Europe. The reason for this is that the WHO is dominated by technical experts who advocate 'One Health' – a twenty-first-century rebranding and expanding of the 'selective primary health care' model. Health surveillance, including global information sharing, as well as a focus on veterinary medicine (zoonosis), are two key aspects of the 'One Health' model. Thus, in the spring of 2005, the maps revealed that cases of avian influenza caused by the H5N1 virus were present first in Southeast Asia and then in China. A second and much worse epidemic than SARS was forecast – a pandemic that would rival the deaths of 1918 – and a worldwide panic ensued. Yet, of course, it was not avian influenza or East Asia that was the origin in 2009: instead it was Mexico, far from the origin of SARS or avian influenza, and the virus appeared first in domesticated pigs, who rarely fly across national boundaries. 'Swine flu' was officially declared a 'pandemic' on 11 June 2009 and caused as many as 500,000 deaths globally.

Yet people who had H1N1 felt their lives were much more at risk, were seen as putting others at risk, and experienced their illness as much more terrifying than if they had had 'normal' influenza. Headlines such as 'SPL Star's Swine Flu Terror as His Little Girl Stops Breathing' from Scotland were typical.[28] Panic was both reflected and generated in such coverage. A mother stated that after her son was diagnosed, 'I couldn't believe it at first. Then I started panicking and reading everything I could find about swine flu.'[29] And first-hand accounts recorded the panic too. Amy McAlister, fourteen, of Potomac, Maryland, wrote: 'I went to the doctor when it hit 103. He did a rapid test. He said he was pretty sure it was swine flu . . . Oh, my God. At first, I thought, "Am I gonna die?"'[30] Her reaction seems not unreasonable given the media coverage.

Perhaps we undersell the dangers of the annual influenza and dismiss it as merely 'like a bad cold', as was done with COVID-19, even though tens of thousands of people die from it each year. Yet H1N1 was not the promised epidemic killer that we had been carefully trained over and over again during the past decades to expect. Such a situation stirs many qualities and emotions to create an illness, not in the sense of inventing it, but in the sense of shaping our experience of it. The 2009 H1N1 influenza turned out not to be equivalent to 1918. But even though it was not as deadly as Spanish flu, in 2020 COVID-19 did indeed begin to replicate the dangers of 1918 to a greater extent than 2009 H1N1 had done. The link between the measures taken to ameliorate the 2020 pandemic and the resistance to them may well be understood through the anxiety that all such threats cause:

Social distancing measures (e.g., keeping six feet apart, wearing masks and gloves) have highlighted the psychological need for social interaction and have uncovered deep feelings of isolation and distress. At the same time, these measures have also revealed reckless behaviors by some Americans who refuse to abide by these health protections. These actions are likely motivated by feelings of entitlement and invincibility. Together, they underscore the current, anti-communitarian strain evident in much of American society.[31]

In 2009 the power of the threat and the attendant panic was real; the epidemic, in the sense of a global threat to life, was not. Margaret Chan and the WHO recognized the politics of the pandemic and rethought its overall political impact on the global economy and global health. But the effect of relabelling a disease as an epidemic or a pandemic in terms of its impact on the individual who becomes ill is also important. And that we must also consider when we label a disease epidemic or pandemic. In 2020 the initial hesitancy to use the word 'pandemic' may well have had its roots in the experiences of 2009. The reality, however, meant that the fear engendered was real and its denial – in the United States, in the UK, in Brazil, in Mexico – led to mass deaths and social dislocation unmatched since 1918–19. The anxiety triggered in all settings the sort of response, that, if it had been 2009, would have been considered overstated.[32] As we have said over and over again in this study, words matter because the emotions they generate have an impact on action. Words have histories, words change our world, making clear whom to blame and whom to absolve from blame. For we know, in our heart of hearts, who is ultimately responsible for our fear. 'I know who caused COVID-19. THEY did.'

REFERENCES

PREFACE: IN TIMES OF STRESS

1 Carol Midgley, 'I Am Writing This in My Silver-lined 5G-resistant Knickers – and You?' *The Times* (London), 8 April 2020, at www.thetimes.co.uk.
2 Neena Satija, '"I do regret being there": Simone Gold, Noted Hydroxychloroquine Advocate, Was Inside the Capitol During the Riot', *Washington Post*, 12 January 2021, at www.washingtonpost.com.

1 XENOPHOBIA AND COVID-19

1 ''Ηρξατο δὲ τὸ μὲν πρῶτον, ὡς λέγεται, ἐξ Αἰθιοπίας τῆς ὑπὲρ Αἰγύπτου, ἔπειτα δὲ καὶ ἐς Αἴγυπτον καὶ Λιβύην κατέβη καὶ ἐς 2τὴν βασιλέως γῆν τὴν πολλήν.' Thucydides, *History of the Peloponnesian War*, vol. I, ed. and trans. C. F. Smith. Loeb Classical Library 108 (Cambridge, MA, 1919), p. 242. See Clifford Orwin, 'Stasis and Plague: Thucydides on the Dissolution of Society', *Journal of Politics*, 50 (1988), pp. 831–47, and Helen King and Jo Brown, 'Thucydides and the Plague', in *A Handbook to the Reception of Thucydides* (Chichester, 2014), ed. Neville Morley and Christine Lee, pp. 447–73. Ned Lebow's work on Thucydides and Greek tragedy frames the argument that this reference should not be taken as 'historical' in our contemporary academic sense but as a continuation of the image of the 'African' in Attic culture. Richard Ned Lebow, *The Tragic Vision of Politics* (Cambridge, 2003), pp. 20ff.
2 As general background on the history of pandemics see John M. Barry, *The Great Influenza: The Story of the Deadliest Plague in History* (New York, 2005); Mark Davis and Davina Lohm, *Pandemics, Publics, and Narrative* (Oxford, 2020); Richard J. Evans, *Death in Hamburg: Society and Politics in the Cholera Years, 1830–1910* (Oxford, 1987); J. N. Hays, *Epidemics and Pandemics: Their Impacts on Human History* (Santa Barbara, CA, 2005); Mark Honigsbaum, *The Pandemic Century:*

One Hundred Years of Panic, Hysteria, and Hubris (New York, 2020); Damir Huremović, ed., *Psychiatry of Pandemics: A Mental Health Response to Infection Outbreak* (Cham, 2019); Christian W. McMillen, *Pandemics: A Very Short Introduction* (Oxford, 2016); Charles E. Rosenberg, *Explaining Epidemics* (Cambridge, 1992); Frank M. Snowden, *Epidemics and Society: From the Black Death to the Present* (New Haven, CT, 2019); Sheldon J. Watts, *Epidemics and History: Disease, Power, and Imperialism* (New Haven, CT, 1997).

3 G. C. Gee, M. J. Ro and A. W. Rimoin, 'Seven Reasons to Care About Racism and COVID-19 and Seven Things to Do to Stop It', *American Journal of Public Health*, 110 (2020), pp. 954–56.

4 We are grateful to George Makari for having allowed us to read the penultimate draft of his *Of Fear and Strangers: A History of Xenophobia* (New York, 2021), prior to publication.

5 Sander L. Gilman and J. M. Thomas, *Are Racists Crazy? How Prejudice, Racism, and Antisemitism Became Markers of Insanity* (New York, 2016; paperback 2018).

6 Rodolfo Lanciani, 'The Archaeological Budget of Rome for 1908', *The Athenaeum* (London) 4246 (13 March 1909), p. 325. On theories of xenophobia see Oksksana Yukushko, *Modern Day Xenophobia: Critical, Historical and Theoretical Perspectives* (Cham, Switzerland, 2018).

7 Sigmund Freud, 'Group Psychology and the Analysis of the Ego (1921)', in *The Standard Edition of the Complete Psychological Works of Sigmund Freud*, ed. James Strachey, vol. XVIII (1920–1922): *Beyond the Pleasure Principle, Group Psychology and Other Works* (London, 1953), pp. 65–144, here p. 100.

8 W. J. Wiersinga et al., 'Pathophysiology, Transmission, Diagnosis, and Treatment of Coronavirus Disease 2019 (COVID-19): A Review', JAMA, CCCXXIV/8 (2020), pp. 782–93.

9 Mary Douglas, *Risk and Blame: Essays in Cultural Theory* (New York, 1992), p. 34.

10 Leon F. Seltzer, 'COVID-19 Hate Crimes: Anger > Indignation > Hatred > Revenge: It's Vital to Fully Appreciate Why Asian American Hate Crimes Are on the Rise', *Psychology Today* (20 April 2020), at www.psychologytoday.com.

11 See Lucius Outlaw, 'Toward a Critical Theory of "Race"', in *Anatomy of Racism*, ed. David Theo Goldberg (Minneapolis, MN, 1992), pp. 58–82, as well as David Theo Goldberg, 'The Social Formation of Racist Discourse', in *Anatomy of Racism*, ed. Goldberg, pp. 295–318.

12 Mark Snyder et al., 'Social Perception and Interpersonal Behavior:

On the Self-fulfilling Nature of Social Stereotypes', *Journal of Personality and Social Psychology*, xxxv/9 (1977), pp. 656–66; Charles Stangor, 'Content and Application Inaccuracy in Social Stereotyping', in *Stereotype Accuracy*, ed. Y. T. Lee et al. (Washington, DC, 1995), pp. 275–92.

13 A. David Napier, 'Rethinking Vulnerability through Covid-19', *Anthropology Today*, 36 (June 2020), pp. 1–2.

14 Historically see C.-E.A. Winslow, 'The Untilled Fields of Public Health', *Science*, LI/1306 (1920), pp. 23–33.

15 Nathaniel Hupert, 'Modeling Pandemics; or, How Mathematics Changes the World', in 'Time of Plague: The History and Social Consequences of Lethal Epidemic Disease: COVID-19 Edition', *Social Research*, 87 (2020), pp. 253–6.

16 David Kindig and Greg Stoddart, 'What is Population Health?' *American Journal of Public Health*, 93 (2003), pp. 380–83.

17 David B. Nash et al., *Population Health: Creating a Culture of Wellness*, 2nd edn (Burlington, MA, 2016).

18 Alexandra King, 'Poor Health Literacy: A "Hidden" Risk Factor', *Nature Reviews Cardiology*, VII/9 (2010), pp. 473–4.

19 Benedict Anderson, *Imagined Communities: Reflections on the Origin and Spread of Nationalism* (London, 1983), p. 19.

20 Ibid., p. 47.

21 William Bloom, *Personal Identity, National Identity, and International Relations* (Cambridge, 1999), p. 52.

22 Ibid., p. 74.

23 Johann Gottfried Herder, *Outlines of a Philosophy of the History of Man*, trans. T. Churchill (London, 1800), p. 658.

24 G. Bateson et al., 'A Note on the Double Bind', *Family Process*, 2 (1962), pp. 154–61, here, p. 154.

25 See Sander L. Gilman, 'AIDS and Syphilis: The Representation of the Individual Living with Disease', *October*, 43 (1987), pp. 87–108; 'Placing the Blame for Devastating Disease', *Social Research*, 55 (1988), pp. 361–78 (with Dorothy Nelkin); 'The Stigma of Disease: 1000 Years', *The Lancet: Millennium Review*, 354 (2000), p. 15; 'Some Weighty Thoughts on Dieting and Epidemics', *The Lancet*, 371 (3 May 2008), pp. 1498–1500; 'Human Papillomavirus, Abstinence, and the Other Risks', *The Lancet*, 373 (25 April 2009), pp. 1420–21; 'Moral Panic and Pandemics', *The Lancet*, 375 (29 May 2010), pp. 1866–7.

26 Freud, 'Group Psychology and the Analysis of the Ego', p. 68.

27 Ibid., p. 63.

28 John Muller, 'Lacan's Mirror Stage', *Psychoanalytic Inquiry*, 5 (1985), pp. 233–52, here 233.

29 Sigmund Freud, 'Civilization and Its Discontents', in *The Standard Edition of the Complete Psychological Works of Sigmund Freud*, ed. James Strachey, vol. XXI (1927–31): *The Future of an Illusion, Civilization and Its Discontents, and Other Works* (London, 1953), pp. 57–146, here p. 103.

30 Françoise Hértier, 'The Symbolics of Incest and Its Prohibition', trans. John Leavitt, in *Between Belief and Transgression: Structuralist Essays in Religion, History, and Myth*, ed. Michel Izard et al. (Chicago, IL, 1982), pp. 152–79.

31 S. Lim et al., 'Face Masks and Containment of COVID-19: Experience from South Korea', *Journal of Hospital Infection*, CVI/1 (2020), pp. 206–7. DOI: 10.1016/j.jhin.2020.06.017. On the implications within such cultures of mask-wearing see Adam Burgess and Mitsutoshi Horii, 'Risk, Ritual and Health Responsibilisation: Japan's "Safety Blanket" of Surgical Face Mask-wearing', *Sociology of Health and Illness*, XXXIV/8 (2012), pp. 1184–98. On masking in the present pandemic see Lindsey Grubbs and Gail Geller, 'Masks in Medicine: Metaphors and Morality', *Journal of Medical Humanities*, 42 (in press, March 2021). doi:.org/10.1007/s10912-020-09676-w.

32 Keith Bradsher, 'A Deadly Virus on Its Mind, Hong Kong Covers Its Face', *New York Times* (31 March 2003), at www.nytimes.com.

33 'Ce qui est commun à toutes les épidémies c'est la recherche des responsables', interview with Anne-Marie Moulin, *Mediapart* (17 March 2020), at www.mediapart.fr.

34 Daniel Kahneman and Amos Tversky, 'Prospect Theory: An Analysis of Decision under Risk', *Econometrica*, XLVII/2 (1979), pp. 263–91.

35 Daniel Kahneman and Amos Tversky, 'Support Theory: A Non-extensional Representation of Subjective Probability', *Psychological Review*, CI/4 (1994), pp. 547–67.

36 See Peter Bernstein, *Against the Gods: The Remarkable Story of Risk* (New York, 1996).

37 Daniel Kahneman, *Thinking, Fast and Slow* (New York, 2011), pp. 168–9.

38 Tedros Adhanom Ghebreyesus, 'Speech of the Director-General, World Health Organization, Munich Security Conference' (15 February 2020), at www.who.int.

39 Corey Williams, 'US Shootings, Killings Spike in COVID-19 Era', *Associate Press News*, 30 December 2020, at www.apnews.com.

40 John Elster, *Ulysses and the Sirens: Studies in Rationality and Irrationality* (Cambridge, 1998); *Ulysses Unbound: Studies in Rationality, Precommitment, and Constraints* (Cambridge, 2000) and John Elser and Nicolas Herpin, eds, *The Ethics of Medical Choice* (London, 1994).

41 Xingru Chen and Feng Fu, 'Imperfect Vaccine and Hysteresis', *Proceedings of the Royal Society* B286 (13 December 2018).

42 Richard J. Evans, *Death in Hamburg: Society and Politics in the Cholera Years, 1830–1910* (Oxford, 1987).

43 'Works on Epidemic Cholera in India', *Quarterly Journal of Medical Sciences* (Madras), 12 (1868), p. 209.

44 Mark Harrison, *Public Health in British India Anglo-Indian Preventive Medicine, 1859–1914* (Cambridge, 1994), p. 132.

45 *Correspondence Respecting the Sanitary Convention Signed at Dresden on 15 April 1893* (London, 1893), p. 34.

46 Lauren Frayer, 'Hindu Nationalists Blame Muslims for India's COVID-19 Crisis', NPR (16 April 2020), at www.npr.org.

47 Gu Yuzhou, Jianyun Lu and Zhicong Yang, 'Pilgrimage and COVID-19: The Risk Among Returnees from Muslim Countries', *International Journal of Infectious Diseases*, 95 (2020), pp. 457–8.

48 Goleen Samari, 'Islamophobia and Public Health in the United States', *American Journal of Public Health*, 106 (2016), pp. 1920–25.

49 A. David Napier, 'Epidemics and Xenophobia; or, Why Xenophilia Matters', *Social Research*, 84 (Spring 2017), pp. 59–81, here p. 60.

50 Two recent studies have proven important in understanding the spread of such views in 2020: Talia Lavin, *Culture Warlords: My Journey into the Dark Web of White Supremacy* (New York, 2020), and Angela Nagle, *Kill All Normies: Online Culture Wars from 4Chan and Tumblr to Trump and the Alt-right* (New York, 2017).

2 CHINA, WUHAN AND RACE

1 Frank Lentz, 'The World's Ancient Porcelain Center', *National Geographic Magazine*, 38 (November, 1920), p. 391. See Larissa N. Heinrich, *The Afterlife of Images: Translating the Pathological Body between China and the West* (Durham, NC, 2008).

2 See Howard Markel and Alexandra Minna Stern, 'The Foreignness of Germs: The Persistent Association of Immigrants and Disease in American Society', *Milbank Quarterly*, 80 (2002), pp. 757–88, as well as Alexandre I. R. White, 'Global Risks, Divergent Pandemics: Contrasting Responses to Bubonic Plague and Smallpox in 1901

Cape Town', *Social Science History*, 42 (2018), pp. 135–58 and her 'Epidemic Orientalism: Social Construction and the Global Management of Infectious Disease', dissertation, Boston University (2018).

3 On eugenics, disease, and the politics of the 'Yellow Peril' see John Kuo Wei Tchen and Dylan Yeats, eds, *Yellow Peril! An Archive of Anti-Asian Fear* (London, 2014), pp. 285ff, and Karen Shimakawa, *National Abjection: The Asian American Body Onstage* (Durham, NC, 2002), pp. 236–41. For the Yellow Peril discourse in European scientific racism see Joseph Arthur De Gobineau, *Oeuvres*, ed. J. Gaulmier et al., 3 vols (Paris, 1983–7), pp. 3: xl, xlvi-xlvii; Ludwig Schemann, *Gobineaus Rassenwerk. Aktenstücke und Betrachtungen zur Geschichte und Kritik des Essai sur l'inégalité des races humaines* (Stuttgart, 1910).

4 *Canada, Report of the Royal Commission on Chinese Immigration* (Ottawa, 1885), p. 128.

5 Nayan Shah, *Contagious Divides: Epidemics and Race in San Francisco's Chinatown* (Berkeley, CA, 2001).

6 Justin A. Chen and Emily Zhang, 'Potential Impact of COVID-19-related Racial Discrimination on the Health of Asian Americans', *American Journal of Public Health*, CX/11 (2020), pp. 1624–7.

7 Shuang Geng, '2020年2月19日外交部发言人耿爽主持网上例行记者会' [Foreign Ministry Spokesperson Geng Shuang Holds Online Routine Press Conference], *Foreign Ministry of the People's Republic of China* (19 February 2020), at www.fmprc.gov.cn.

8 Harry Zhang, 'Headline Echoes the Worst of Old China's Exploitation', *Wall Street Journal*, 7 February 2020, at www.wsj.com.

9 S. O. Cheng, 'Xenophobia Due to the Coronavirus Outbreak – a Letter to the Editor in Response to "The Socio-economic Implications of the Coronavirus Pandemic (COVID-19): A Review"', *International Journal of Surgery*, 79 (2020), pp. 13–14.

10 This was highly symbolic as it was here the Wuchang uprising broke out that would lead to the revolution that overthrew thousands of years of imperial rule. Subsequently China would become the first modern republic in Asia, depicted in the Chinese history books as the nation's first step on the path to regain its worth and power.

11 Zhou Xun, *The People's Health: Health Intervention and Delivery in Mao's China, 1949–1983* (Montreal, 2020).

12 Robert Zaretsky, 'An Unwilling Guide: Camus's *The Plague*', *In Time*

of Plague: The History and Social Consequences of Lethal Epidemic Disease: COVID-19 Edition, Social Research, 87 (2020), pp. 297–300.

13 On the trial and sentencing see Vivian Wang, 'Chinese Citizen Journalist Sentenced to 4 Years for Covid Reporting', *New York Times*, 28 December 2020, at www.nytimes.com.

14 Fang Fang, *Wuhan Diary: Dispatches from a Quarantined City*, trans. Michael Berry (New York, 2020).

15 Michael Standaert, '"Even mourning is said to shame China": Women of Wuhan Fight to Be Heard', *The Guardian*, 20 January 2021, at www.theguardian.com.

16 Associate Press, 'How China Blocked WHO and Chinese Scientist Early in Coronavirus Outbreak', *NBC News*, 2 June 2020, at www.nbcnews.com.

17 截至1月13日24时新型冠状病毒肺炎疫情最新情况 [The Latest Updates of the Novel Coronavirus Pneumonia Epidemic as of Midnight on 13 January], 14 January 2021, at www.nhc.gov.cn.

18 Sarah Boseley, 'China Blocks Entry to WHO team studying COVID's Origins', *The Guardian*, 2 January 2021, at www.theguardian.com.

19 'Foreign Ministry Spokesperson Hua Chunying's Regular Press Conference on 7 January 2021', at http://ie.china-embassy.org/eng; http://ie.china-embassy.org/eng, accessed 15 January 2021.

20 Javier C. Hernández, 'Two Members of WHO Team on Trail of Virus Are Denied Entry to China', *New York Times*, 13 January 2021, at www.nytimes.com.

21 Matthew Campbell and Philip Sherwell, 'WHO in Wuhan: The Covidhunters Will Trudge Wherever They Are Allowed', *The Times* (London), 17 January 2021, at www.thetimes.co.uk.

22 S. Duan et al. 'Seroprevalence and Asymptomatic Carrier Status of SARS-COV-2 in Wuhan City and Other Places of China', *PLoS Neglected Tropical Diseases*, xv/1 (2021): e0008975, DOI: 10.1371/journal.pntd.0008975.

23 Gerald L. Geison, *The Private Science of Louis Pasteur* (Princeton, NJ, 1995); Susan E. Lederer, *Human Experimentation in America before the Second World War* (Baltimore, MD, 1995).

24 James Gorman, 'A WHO Researcher on his Trip to China Seeking Origins of the Virus', *New York Times*, 14 February 2021, at www.nytimes.com.

25 Javier C. Hernández and James Gorman, 'On WHO Trip, China Refused to Hand Over Important Data', *New York Times*, 12 February 2021, at www.nytimes.com. See also Peipei Liu et al., 'Cold-chain

Transportation in the Frozen Food Industry May Have Caused a Recurrence of COVID-19 Cases in Destination: Successful Isolation of SARS-CoV-2 Virus from the Imported Frozen Cod Package Surface', *Biosafety and Health*, 2 (2020), pp. 199–201.

26 "The Birth of WHO: Interview with Dr Szeming Sze', *World Health Forum* (28–29 May 1989), pp. 28–9.

27 Martin Enserink, 'SARS Linked to Wild Animals', *Science*, 23 May 2003, at www.sciencemag.org.

28 Diana J. Bell, Scott Robertson and Paul R. Hunter, 'Animal Origins of SARS Coronavirus: Possible Links with the International Trade in Small Carnivores', in *SARS: A Case Study in Emerging Infections*, ed. Angela McLean et al. (Oxford, 2005), pp. 51–60. See also Jacalyn Duffin and Arthur Sweetman, eds, *SARS in Context: Memory, History, Policy* (Montreal, 2006).

29 'Introduction', in Arthur Kleinman and James L. Watson, eds, *SARS in China: Prelude to a Pandemic?* (Stanford, CA, 2003), pp. 17–30, here p. 17.

30 Pete Davies, *Catching Cold: 1918's Forgotten Tragedy and the Scientific Hunt for the Virus that Caused It* (London, 1999), as well as J. S. Malik Peiris and Yi Guan, 'Confronting SARS: A View from Hong Kong', in *SARS*, ed. McLean et al., pp. 35–40.

31 Hong Zhang, 'Making Light of the Dark Side', in *SARS in China*, ed. Kleinman and Watson, pp. 148–70, here p. 152.

32 Ibid., p. 164.

33 Alexander Michie, *The Englishman in China During the Victorian Era, as Illustrated in the Career of Sir Rutherford Alcock* (London, 1890), pp. 127–8 on pheasant shooting in China.

34 Claude Fischler, 'Food, Self and Identity', *Social Science Information*, 27 (1988), pp. 275–93.

35 Katie Shepherd, 'John Cornyn Criticized Chinese for Eating Snakes. He Forgot About the Rattlesnake Roundups Back in Texas', *Washington Post*, 19 March 2020, at www.washingtonpost.com.

36 'Letter of Aristeas', ed. R. H. Charles (Oxford, 1913), vv. 143–58, at www.ccel.org.

37 William Loader, "Not as the Gentiles": Sexual Issues at the Interface between Judaism and Its Greco-Roman World', *Religions*, 9 (2018), p. 258, at DOI: 10.3390/rel9090258.

38 Mary Douglas, 'The Abominations of Leviticus', *Purity and Danger: An Analysis of the Concept of Pollution and Taboo* (New York, 1966; repr. 1998), pp. 42–58. See also her 2002 introduction to the reprint of *Purity and Danger* (pp. xi, 1), which abandoned this earlier

work on the abominations that stressed their symbolic boundary maintenance. She had argued that ambiguity, a central concept in our present study, led to the exclusion of certain animals from consumption. On her rereading she stressed that animals that were excluded were those also excluded from sacrifice at the Temple. See T. M. Lemos, 'The Universal and the Particular: Mary Douglas and the Politics of Impurity', *Journal of Religion*, LXXXIX/2 (2009), pp. 236–51. That her earlier approach remains fruitful; see Patrick Brown 'Studying COVID-19 in Light of Critical Approaches to Risk and Uncertainty: Research Pathways, Conceptual Tools, and Some Magic from Mary Douglas', *Health, Risk and Society*, XXII/1 (2020), pp. 1–14.

39 Christoph Riedweg, *Pythagoras: His Life, Teaching, and Influence*, trans. Stephen Rendell (Ithaca, NY, 2005), pp. 70–71.

40 For further reading, see David M. Freidenreich, *Foreigners and Their Food: Constructing Otherness in Jewish, Christian, and Islamic Law* (Berkeley, CA, 2011).

41 John de Marignolli, 'Recollections of Easter Travel (1338–53)', in *Great Travel Stories from All Nations*, ed. Elizabeth D'Oyley (London, 1932), pp. 665–6.

42 Quoted by Henry Yule, ed. and trans., *Cathay and the Way Thither, Being a Collection of Medieval Notices of China* (London, 1866), vol. I, p. 107.

43 J. Gernet, *Daily Life in China on the Eve of the Mongol Invasion*, trans. H. M. Wright (Stanford, CA, 1962), p. 142, n.49.

44 A remarkable account of the culture, mystery and anxiety attendant on eel consumption is Patrik Svensson, *The Book of Eels: Our Enduring Fascination with the Most Mysterious Creature in the Natural World*, trans. Agnes Broome (New York, 2020).

45 James Lind, *An Essay on Diseases Incidental to Europeans, in Hot Climates: with the Method of Preventing their fatal Consequences* (London, 1768).

46 Hans Staden, *The True History of his Captivity*, ed. and trans. Michael Letts [1557] (New York, 1929), cited in John H. Elliot, 'Renaissance Europe and America: A Blunted Impact?' in *First Images of America: The Impact of the New World on the Old*, ed. Fredi Chiappelli, Michael J. B. Allen and Robert Louis Benson (Berkeley, Los Angeles, London, 1976), p. 20. See also Nancy Stepan, *Picturing Tropical Nature* (Ithaca, NY, 2001).

47 Rudyard Kipling, *The Works of Rudyard Kipling: Plain Tales from the Hills* [1888] (Boston, MA, 1899), p. 53.

48 Zhou, *The People's Health*, p. 54.

49 Hans Kruuk, *Otters: Ecology, Behaviour and Conservation* (Oxford, 2006).

50 J. Blancou and F. X. Meslin, 'Brefs rappels sur l'histoire des zoonoses', *Revue scientifique et technique*, 19 (2000), pp. 15–22.

51 中国疾控中心在武汉华南海鲜市场检出大量新型冠状病毒 [China CDC Detects a Large Number of New Coronaviruses in Wuhan South China Seafood Market], 27 January 2020, www.chinacdc.cn.

52 Amy Qin and Javier C. Hernández, 'A Year After Wuhan, China Tells a Tale of Triumph (and No Mistakes)', *New York Times*, 10 January 2021, at www.nytimes.com.

53 Raymond Zhong, Paul Mozur, Jeff Kao and Aaron Krolik, 'No "Negative" News: How China Censored the Coronavirus', *New York Times*, 19 December 2020, at www.nytimes.com.

54 Yingchun Zeng and Yan Zhen, 'RETRACTED: Chinese Medical Staff Request International Medical Assistance in Fighting Against COVID 19', *The Lancet* (24 February 2020), at www.thelancet.com.

55 On the complex legal and cultural contexts of xenophobia in the Asian pandemic see Victor V. Ramraj, ed., COVID-19 *in Asia: Law and Policy Contexts* (Oxford, 2020).

56 See Frank Dikötter, Zhou Xun and Lars Laamann, *Narcotic Culture: A Social History of Drug Consumption in Modern China* (London and Chicago, 2018); Julia Lovell, *The Opium War: Drugs, Dreams, and the Making of China* (London, 2011).

57 Zhou, *The People's Health*, pp. 279–85.

58 James Palmer, 'The "Phase One" Trade Deal Is Still Hypothetical', *Newstex Blogs Foreign Policy*, 15 January 2020, at https://advance. lexis.com.

59 '"Coronavirus" Sprayed on Japanese Restaurant in Paris', *Straits Times*, 22 February 2020, at www.straitstimes.com.

60 Manuela Pellegrino, 'COVID-19: The "Invisible Enemy" and Contingent Racism', *Anthropology Today*, 26 (2020), pp. 19–21, here 20.

61 'Stop AAPI Hate National Report 3.19.20–8.5.20', www. asianpacificpolicyandplanningcouncil.org, accessed 3 February 2021. Updated 9 February 2021: https://secureservercdn. net/104.238.69.231/a1w.90d.myftpupload.com/wp-content/ uploads/2021/02/Press-Statement-re_-Bay-Area-Elderly- Incidents-2.9.2021-1.pdf.

62 Tyler T. Reny and Matt A. Barreto, 'Xenophobia in the Time of Pandemic: Othering, Anti-Asian Attitudes, and COVID-19',

Politics, Groups, and Identities (28 May 2020), in press, DOI: 10.1080/21565503.2020.1769693); Stephen W. Pan, Gordon C. Shen, Chuncheng Liu, Jenny H. His, 'Coronavirus Stigmatization and Psychological Distress Among Asians in the United States', *Ethnicity and Health*, XXVI/1 (2021), pp. 110–25.

63 Mark Townsend and Noshee Iqbal, 'Far Right Using Coronavirus as Excuse to Attack Chinese and South East Asians, Police Say', *The Guardian*, 29 August 2020, at www.theguardian.com.

64 Frank Dikötter, *The Discourse of Race in Modern China*, revd edn (Oxford, 2015). See also Frank Dikötter, *Imperfect Conceptions: Medical Knowledge, Birth Defects, and Eugenics in China* (London, 1998).

65 Zang Qian, 'African Media Attends Seminar on "Chinese Dream" and "African Dream"', *People's Daily Online*, 18 September 2013, at http://en.people.cn.

66 Todd Samuel Presner, '"Clear Heads, Solid Stomachs, and Hard Muscles": Max Nordau and the Aesthetics of Jewish Regeneration', *Modernism/Modernity*, 10 (2003), pp. 269–96.

67 Yuehtsen Juliette Chung, *Struggle for National Survival: Eugenics in Sino-Japanese Contexts, 1896–1945* (New York and London, 2002), pp. 72–85; Dikötter, *Imperfect Conceptions*, pp. 64–104.

68 Pamela Kyle Crossley, *A Translucent Mirror: History and Identity in Qing Imperial Ideology* (Berkeley, CA, 2000).

69 Rong Ma, 'Ethnic Relations in Contemporary China: Cultural Tradition and Ethnic Policies Since 1949', *Policy and Society*, XXV/1 (2006), pp. 85–108, DOI: 10.1016/S1449-4035(06)70128-x.

70 Zhou Xun, 'Discourse of Disability in Modern China', *Pattern and Prejudice*, XXXVI/1 (2002), pp. 104–12, here, 110–12.

71 Zhou Min, Shabnam Shenasi and Tao Xu, 'Chinese Attitudes toward African Migrants in Guangzhou, China', *International Journal of Sociology*, XLVI/2 (2016), pp. 141–61.

72 '潘慶林：從嚴從速全力以赴解決廣東省非洲黑人群居的問題', [Pan Qinglin, 'Urgently and Stringently Resolve the Problem of the Black African Population Living in Herds in Guangdong], https://chinadigitaltimes.net, accessed 19 December 2020.

73 'China: Covid-19 Discrimination Against Africans', *Human Rights Watch* (5 May 2020), at www.hrw.org.

74 *Report of the Canadian Royal Commission on Chinese and Japanese Immigration*, Royal Commission on Chinese Immigration: VII. Sessional Papers, No. 54 (Ottawa, 1902), p. 277.

3 COVID-19 IN ULTRA-ORTHODOX JEWISH COMMUNITIES

1 We are citing here what has become the classic study, Barbara
   Tuchman, *A Distant Mirror: The Calamitous 14th Century* (New York,
   1978), p. 109. See more recently Ron Barkaï, 'Jewish Treatises on the
   Black Death (1350–1500): A Preliminary Study', in *Medicine from the
   Black Death to the French Disease*, ed. Roger French, Jon Arrizabalaga,
   Andrew Cunningham and Luis García-Ballester (London 1998),
   pp. 6–25; Anna Foa, *The Jews of Europe after the Black Death*
   (Berkeley and Los Angeles, CA, 2000); Cordelia Heß, 'Jews and the
   Black Death in 14th century Prussia', in *Fear and Loathing in the
   North: Jews and Muslims in Medieval Scandinavia and the Baltic Region*,
   ed. Cordelia Heß and Jonathan Adams (Berlin, 2015), pp. 109–25;
   Klaus Bergdolt, 'Die Pest und die Juden. Mythen, Fakten, Topoi',
   Aschkenas: Zeitschrift für Geschichte und Kultur der Juden, 29 (2019),
   pp. 43–62.
2 Salo W. Baron, *A Social and Religious History of the Jews*, vol. XI: *Late
   Middle Ages and Era of European Expansion (1200–1650), Citizen or
   Alien Conjurer*, 2nd edn (New York, 1967), p. 160.
3 Naomi E. Pasachoff and Robert J. Littman, eds, *A Concise History
   of the Jewish People* (Lanham, MD, 2005), p. 154. 'However, Jews
   regularly ritually washed and bathed, and their abodes were slightly
   cleaner than their Christian neighbors. Consequently, when
   the rat and the flea brought the Black Death, Jews, with better
   hygiene, suffered less severely.' One of the authors of this book
   has spent a great deal of effort trying to contextualize these claims
   about Jewish immunity from infectious diseases which began in
   allopathic medicine in the nineteenth century and were attributed
   to claims about Jewish hygiene practices or to racial predisposition.
   Neither were true. See Sander L. Gilman, 'Tuberculosis as a Test
   Case', in his *Franz Kafka: The Jewish Patient* (New York, 1995), pp.
   169–228 as well as Adrienne Denoyelles, '"Peculiar Resistance":
   Tuberculosis, Identity and Conflict among Jewish Physicians
   in Early-twentieth-century America', *American Jewish History*,
   C/3 (2016), pp. 349–77, DOI:10.1353/ajh.2016.0037. As early as the
   nineteenth century, historians of medicine refuted the very notion
   that Jews were 'immune' to the Black Death; see Justus Hecker's
   first comprehensive study of the Black Death in 1832. It was clear
   that the Jews suffered from the pandemic as greatly as their non-
   Jewish neighbours. Indeed, Hecker notes that in communities where
   the Jews had been expelled such as Magdeburg and Leipzig, the

blame for the plague was laid at the feet of the grave-diggers, not the Jews. Justus Friedrich Carl Hecker, *Der schwarze Tod im vierzehnten Jahrhundert: Nach Quellen für Ärzte und gebildete Nichtärzte bearbeitet* (Berlin, 1832), pp. 52–3. See also Joseph Jacobs, *Studies in Jewish Statistics: Social, Vital and Anthropomorphic* (London, 1891), pp. viii–ix for a number of sources and, more recently, Dean Phillip Bell, *Jews in the Early Modern World* (Lanham, MD, 2008), p. 41 on Jewish demography during the plague.

4 On the instrumentalization of the Black Death in the history of antisemitism see Nico Voigtländer and Hans-Joachim Voth, 'Persecution Perpetuated: The Medieval Origins of Anti-Semitic Violence in Nazi Germany', *Quarterly Journal of Economics*, 127 (2012), pp. 1339–92, and Theresa Finley and Mark Koyama, 'Plague, Politics, and Pogroms: The Black Death, the Rule of Law, and the Persecution of Jews in the Holy Roman Empire', *Journal of Law and Economics*, 61 (2018), pp. 253–77.

5 Mark Hay, 'How Holocough went from Anti-Semitic Threat to COVID-19 Truther Rallying Cry', *Daily Beast*, 8 September 2020, at www.thedailybeast.com.

6 Jayita Mukhopadhyay, 'Towards a New World', *The Statesman* (10 August 2020), at www.thestatesman.com.

7 Zhou Xun, 'Review of Daniel Chirot and Anthony Reid, eds, *Essential Outsiders: Chinese and Jews in the Modern Transformation of Southeast Asia and Central Europe*', *China Quarterly*, 174 (June 2003), pp. 547–9.

8 See Howard Markel and Alexandra Minna Stern, 'The Foreignness of Germs: The Persistent Association of Immigrants and Disease in American Society', *Milbank Quarterly*, 80 (2002), pp. 757–88; Allan Kraut, 'Foreign Bodies: The Perennial Negotiation over Health and Culture in a Nation of Immigrants', *Journal of American Ethnic History*, XXIII/2 (2004), pp. 3–22; Howard Markel, *Quarantine! East European Jewish Immigrants and the New York City Epidemics of 1892* (Baltimore, MD, 1997).

9 Sean Clare, 'Losing a "Beacon of Light" of the UK's Ultra-Orthodox Community to Coronavirus', 19 May 2020, at www.bbc.co.uk; Joyce Dalsheim, 'Jewish History Explains Why Some Ultra-Orthodox Communities Defy Coronavirus Restrictions', *The Conversation* (29 April 2020), at https://theconversation.com.

10 Haven Orecchio-Egresitz, 'Orthodox and Hasidic Jews Are Being Scapegoated for the Coronavirus Crisis in a New York Suburb. It's Bringing Decades of Community Controversy to the Surface',

Business Insider (27 May 2020), at www.businessinsider.com.

11 Ibid.

12 Theodor Adorno et al., *The Authoritarian Personality* (New York, 1964), vol. I, p. 71.

13 Oliver Holmes, 'Calls To Seal Off Ultra-Orthodox Areas Add to Israel's Virus Tensions', *The Guardian*, 6 April 2020, at www.theguardian.com.

14 Ilan Rosenberg, 'Israel Seals Off Ultra-Orthodox Town Hit Hard by Coronavirus', *Reuters*, 2 April 2020, at https://fr.reuters.com.

15 Liam Stack, '"Plague on a Biblical Scale": Hasidic Families Hit Hard by Virus', *New York Times*, 21 April 2020, updated 8 October 2020, at www.nytimes.com.

16 Ibid.

17 Liam Stack, 'De Blasio Breaks Up Rabbi's Funeral and Lashes Out Over Virus Distancing', *New York Times*, 28 April 2020, at www.nytimes.com.

18 Joseph Goldstein, 'NYC Warns About Rising Virus Cases in Hasidic Neighborhoods', *New York Times*, 22 September 2020, updated 25 September 2020, at www.nytimes.com.

19 Ibid.

20 Robert McDonald et al., 'Notes from the Field: Measles Outbreaks from Imported Cases in Orthodox Jewish Communities – New York and New Jersey, 2018–2019', MMW: *Morbidity and Mortality Weekly Report*, LXVIII/19 (May 2019), pp. 444–5, EBSCOhost, DOI:10.15585/mmwr.mm6819a4.

21 Tyler Pager, '"Monkey, Rat and Pig DNA": How Misinformation Is Driving the Measles Outbreak Among Ultra-Orthodox Jews', *New York Times*, 9 April 2019, at www.nytimes.com.

22 Jake Offenhartz, 'Orthodox Anti-maskers Crash NYC COVID Outreach, Scream Racial Epithets', *The Gothamist* (25 September 2020), at www.gothamist.com.

23 Goldstein, 'NYC Warns About Rising Virus Cases in Hasidic Neighborhoods'.

24 Liam Stack, 'Backlash Grows in Orthodox Jewish Areas Over Virus Crackdown by Cuomo', *New York Times*, 7 October 2020, updated 8 October 2020, at www.nytimes.com.

25 Teo Armus, 'Brooklyn's Orthodox Jews Burn Masks in Violent Protests as New York Cracks Down on Rising Coronavirus Cases', *Washington Post*, 8 October 2020, at www.washingtonpost.com.

26 Myles Miller, @mylesmill, www.twitter.com/MylesMill/status/1313832787191898113, 7 October 2020.

27 Richard Silverstein., 'At MAGA Rally, Israeli Flag and Neo-Nazis Co-exist Awkwardly', *Newstex Blogs Tikun Olam: Make the World a Better Place*, 8 January 2021, at https://advance.lexis.com.

28 Mallory Simon and Sara Sidner, 'Decoding the Extremist Symbols and Groups at the Capitol Hill Insurrection', *CNN Wire*, 9 January 2021, at https://advance.lexis.com.

29 Jonathan D. Sarna, 'A Scholar of American Anti-Semitism Explains the Hate Symbols Present at the U.S. Capitol', *The Conversation – United States* (8 January 2021), at https://advance.lexis.com.

30 Shira Hanau, 'Orthodox Jewish Trump Supporters Decry Violence, But Not Movement that Fueled It', *Times of Israel*, 7 January 2021, www.timesofisrael.com.

31 Shira Hanau, 'Fur Pelt Rioter Said to Be Son of NY Jewish Judge, Led National Synagogue Group', *Times of Israel*, 7 January 2021, at www.timesofisrael.com.

32 Arutz Sheva Staff, 'Young Israel Condemns "Double Standard" in NY Covid Restrictions', *Arutz Sheva*, 11 October 2020, at https://advance.lexis.com.

33 Elchanan Poupko, 'American Orthodoxy's Political Suicide', *Times of Israel*, 7 January 2021, at https://blogs.timesofisrael.com.

34 Hanau, 'Orthodox Jewish Trump Supporters Decry Violence, But Not Movement that Fueled It'.

35 Rabbi Yosef Blau, 'Orthodox Jewry and President Trump', *The Commentator: Independent Student Newspaper of Yeshiva University*, 22 January 2021, https://yucommentator.org.

36 Gila Jedwab, 'Trusting God to Run His World', *The Five Towns Jewish Times*, 26 June 2020, at www.5tjt.com/jedwab-t.

37 Ronen Bergman, 'How the Pandemic Nearly Tore Israel Apart', *New York Times*, 25 February 2021, at www.nytimes.com.

38 Patrick Kingsley, 'He Is Israel's "Prince of Torah". But to Some, He Is the King of Covid', *New York Times*, 29 January 2021, at www.nytimes.com.

39 Ben Kasstan, '"A Free People, Controlled Only by God": Circulating and Converting Criticism of Vaccination in Jerusalem', *Culture, Medicine, Psychiatry*, 4 February 2021, DOI: 10.1007/s11013-020-09705-2.

40 Danielle Ziri, 'U.S. Chabad Rabbi Fired for Barrage of Anti-vaccine Social Media Posts', *Haaretz*, 3 February 2021, at www.haaretz.com.

41 Shawn Francis Peters, *When Prayer Fails: Faith Healing, Children, and the Law* (New York, 2007), pp. 94–5.

42 Donald G. McNeil Jr, 'Religious Objections to the Measles Vaccine?

Get the Shots, Faith Leaders Say', *New York Times*, 26 April 2019, www.nytimes.com.

43 David M. Halbfinger and Isabel Kershner, 'Israel's Virus Czar Was Making Headway. Then He Tangled with a Key Netanyahu Ally', *New York Times*, 8 September 2020, updated 29 September 2020, at www.nytimes.com.

44 Isabel Kershner, 'Israel to Celebrate Jewish New Year Under a Second Lockdown', *New York Times*, 13 September 2020, updated 18 September 2020, at www.nytimes.com.

45 Times of Israel staff, 'Police Disperse Violent Protesters Yelling "Nazis" in Jerusalem Haredi Area', *Times of Israel*, 14 April 2020, at www.timesofisrael.com.

46 Steve Hendrix and Shira Rubin, 'Israel Is Vaccinating So Fast It's Running Out of Vaccine', *Washington Post*, 4 January 2021, www.washingtonpost.com.

47 Steve Hendrix and Shira Rubin, 'Anger Grows At Israel's Ultra-Orthodox Virus Scofflaws, Threatening Rupture with Secular Jews', *Washington Post*, 9 February 2021, at www.washingtonpost.com.

48 Patrick Kingsley, 'As Ultra-Orthodox Defy Israel's Rules, Virus Exacts a Grim Toll', *New York Times*, 8 February 2021, at www.nytimes.com.

49 Stuti Mishra, '"20,000" Break Rules to Attend Funeral of Orthodox Rabbi as Israel Extends Lockdown', *The Independent*, 31 January 2021, at www.independent.co.uk.

50 'Fresh Clashes in Bnei Brak as Haredi Leaders Blame Police for Violence', *Times of Israel*, 24 January 2021, at www.timesofisrael.com.

51 Ronen Bergman, 'How the Pandemic Nearly Tore Israel Apart', *New York Times*, 25 February 2021, at www.nytimes.com.

52 Helmut Reister, 'Die Stadt untersagt künftig das Tragen von "Judensternen" auf Corona-Demos', *Jüdische Allgemeine*, 11 November 2020, www.juedische-allgemeine.de.

53 Dan Sales, 'Anti-vax Protestors Clash with Police Outside Parliament as Ministers Plunge London into Tier Three', *MailOnline*, 14 December 2020, www.dailymail.co.uk.

54 Isabel Kershner, 'How Israel Became a World Leader in Vaccinating Against Covid-19', *New York Times*, 1 January 2021, www.nytimes.com.

55 'Rabbi Yitzchak Zilberstein: Vaccine Has the Authority of Beis Din and Should Be Taken', *Voz iz Neias?*, 24 December 2020, at https://vosizneias.com.

56 Ben Kasstan, *Making Bodies Kosher: The Politics of Reproduction among Haredi Jews in England* (Oxford, 2019), pp. 231–2.

57 Isabel Kershner and Adam Rasgon, 'After Quick Vaccine Success, Israel Faces New Virus Woes', *New York Times*, 6 January 2021, at www.nytimes.com.

58 Daniel B. Schwartz, *Ghetto: The History of a Word* (Cambridge, MA, 2019).

59 Ibid., p. 38.

60 Ibid., p. 104.

61 Ibid., p. 6.

62 Ibid., p. 52.

63 Ibid., p. 115.

64 Mitchell Duneier, *Ghetto: The Invention of a Place, The History of an Idea* (New York, 2016), pp. 95–107.

65 Amnon Gutman, 'The Coronavirus? Just Follow the Torah. Everything Will Be Alright', *Web24 News*, 7 April 2020, at www.web24.news.

66 Samuel Heilman and Menachem Friedman, *The Rebbe: The Life and Afterlife of Menachem Mendel Schneerson* (Princeton, NJ, 2012).

67 Zach Helfand, '"We Don't Protest": Borough Park's Mask-burning Demonstrators', *New Yorker* (1 November 2020), at www.newyorker.com.

68 'Agudath Israel Statement on Uptick in COVID-19 Cases', https://agudah.org, 30 August 2020.

69 Nathan Jeffay, 'Haredi Health Pioneer: COVID-19 Defiance Fuels Anti-Semitism, Sullies God's Name', *Times of Israel*, 12 October 2020, www.timesofisrael.com.

70 Tara Kavaler, 'Ultra-Orthodox Jews Reject Coronavirus Non-compliance Claims', *The Medialine*, 29 March 2020, at www.themedialine.org.

71 Robert Booth, 'UK Supreme Court Backs Housing Charity's "Jewish Only" Rule', *The Guardian*, 16 October 2020, at www.theguardian.com.

72 Haven Orecchio-Egresitz, 'Orthodox and Haredi Hasidic Jews in a New York Suburb Say They're Scapegoats in the Coronavirus Crisis. The "Othering" Goes Back Decades', *Business Insider: Australia*, 28 May 2020, at www.businessinsider.com.au.

73 Avi Shafran, 'Mayor de Blasio Is No Enemy of Orthodox Jews, But Others Are Vilifying Us', *Jerusalem Post*, 30 April 2020, at www.jpost.com.

74 'A Portrait of American Orthodox Jews: A Further Analysis of the 2013 Survey of U.S. Jews', *Pew Research Center for Religion and Public Life* (26 August 2015), at www.pewforum.org.

75 Dan Zaken, 'Haredim Aren't as Poor as You Think', *The Globes*, 17 December 2018, en.globes.co.il.
76 Personal message, 1 October 2020.
77 Alexandra Levine, 'Faigy Mayer's Brave Life and Shocking Death', *The Forward*, 7 August 2015, at https://forward.com.
78 Isabel Kershner, 'Virus Hastens Exit from Israel's Ultra-Orthodox Community', *New York Times*, 8 February 2021, at www.nytimes.com.
79 Yitz Greenberg, 'Religious Leadership Is Also to Blame for COVID-19 Crisis in Israel', *Jerusalem Post*, 28 September 2020, at www.jpost.com.
80 Shafran, 'Mayor de Blasio Is No Enemy of Orthodox Jews'.
81 Judy Maltz, 'Aliyah and Coronavirus: 24 New Immigrants from U.S. Land in Israel, While Flight from Ethiopia Canceled', *Haaretz*, 19 March 2020, at www.haaretz.com; Adam Rasgon, 'Israel Accepts Ethiopians of Jewish Descent, but Fewer than Promised', *New York Times*, 12 October 2020; updated 5 November 2020, at www.nytimes.com.
82 Orecchio-Egresitz, 'Orthodox and Hasidic Jews Are Being Scapegoated for the Coronavirus Crisis in a New York Suburb'.
83 Sherita Hill Golden, 'Coronavirus in African Americans and Other People of Color', *Johns Hopkins Medicine* (20 April 2020), at www.hopkinsmedicine.org.
84 Loubaba Mamluk and Tim Jones, 'The Impact of Covid-19 on Black, Asian and Minority Ethnic Communities', *National Institute of Health Research Paper*, 20 May 2020, at https://arc-w.nihr.ac.uk.
85 Grey Hutton, 'How a Haredi Community in London Is Coping with Coronavirus', *The Guardian*, 26 May 2020, at www.theguardian.com.
86 'Covid: 400-person Wedding Party in Stamford Hill Broken Up by Police', *BBC News*, 22 January 2021, at www.bbc.com/news.
87 Ellie Jacobs, 'JN Investigation: "For Months They've Broken Every Rule in the Book"', *Jewish Times* (London), 28 January 2021, at https://jewishnews.timesofisrael.com.
88 Isabel Kershner, 'Badly Ill with Coronavirus, Some Ultra-Orthodox in Israel Choose Home Care', *New York Times*, 16 October 2020, www.nytimes.com.
89 Hannah Arendt, *The Origins of Totalitarianism* (San Diego, CA, 1976), p. 34.
90 Ibid., p. 11.
91 Kershner, 'Badly Ill with Coronavirus, Some Ultra-Orthodox in Israel Choose Home Care'.

92 John Locke, *Letter Concerning Toleration* [1689], at www.let.rug.nl.

93 Immanuel Kant, 'On the Question: What Is Enlightenment?', trans. James Schmidt in his *What Is Enlightenment? Eighteenth Century Answers and Twentieth-century Questions* (Berkeley and Los Angeles, CA, 1996), p. 58.

94 Jonathan A. Jacobs, 'Judaism, Pluralism and Public Reason', *Daedalus*, 149 (2020), pp. 169–84, here, 181.

95 Antoon Braeckman, 'The Moral Inevitability of Enlightenment and the Precariousness of the Moment: Reading Kant's *What Is Enlightenment?*', *Review of Metaphysics*, 62 (December 2008), pp. 295–306, here 286.

96 Sander L. Gilman, 'Cosmopolitisme et nomadisme juifs dans l'histoire des idées', in *Juifs d'ailleurs: Diasporas oubliées, identités singulières*, ed. Edith Bruder (Paris, 2020), pp. 369–75.

97 Paul R. Mendes-Flohr and Jehuda Reinharz, eds, *The Jew in the Modern World: A Documentary History* (Detroit, MI, 1995), p. 201.

98 Samson Raphael Hirsch, *Timeless Torah: An Anthology of the Writings of Rabbi Samson Raphael Hirsch*, ed. and trans. Jacob Breuer (New York, 1957), p. 86.

99 Mark Gelber, *Kafka, Zionism, and Beyond* (Tübingen, 2004), p. 38.

100 Sarah Maslin Nir and Sharon Otterman, '15% of Virus Tests Are Positive, and Few Wear Masks in One Orthodox Suburb', *New York Times*, 9 October 2020; updated 13 October 2020, at www.nytimes.com.

101 Myer Siemistycki, 'Contesting Sacred Urban Space: The Case of the *Eruv*', *Journal of International Migration and Integration*, 6 (2005), pp. 255–70.

102 Davina Cooper, 'Talmudic Territory? Space, Law, and Modernist Discourse', *Journal of Law and Society*, 23 (December 1996), pp. 529–48.

103 Leopold Zunz, *Gutachten über die Beschneidung* (Frankfurt am Main, 1844).

104 Jacob Katz, 'The Controversy over the Mezizah: The Unrestricted Execution of the Rite of Circumcision' and 'The Struggle over Preserving the Rite of Circumcision in the First Part of the Nineteenth Century', in his *Divine Law in Human Hands: Case Studies in Halakhic Flexibility* (Jerusalem, 1998), pp. 320–402.

105 Sharon Otterman, 'Board Votes to Regulate Circumcision, Citing Risks', *New York Times*, 13 September 2012, at www.nytimes.com.

106 Ibid.

107 Times of Israel Staff, 'Israel's Chief Rabbinate Backs Metzitzah B'peh Rite', *Times of Israel*, 25 April 2013, at www.timesofisrael.com.

108 Michael M. Grynbaum, 'Mayor de Blasio Is Set to Ease Rules on Circumcision Ritual', *New York Times*, 24 February 2015, at www.nytimes.com.

109 Ibid.

110 Paul Berger 'New Controversial Circumcision Rite Rules: Don't Ask, Don't Tell', *The Forward* (25 September 2015), at https://forward.com.

111 Halbfinger and Kershner, 'Israel's Virus Czar Was Making Headway: Then He Tangled with a Key Netanyahu Ally'.

112 Steve Hendrix, 'Ultra-Orthodox Jews Clash with Secular Israeli Officials Over Coronavirus Measures', *Washington Post*, 5 September 2020, at www.washingtonpost.com.

113 See in this context Sander L. Gilman and Steven T. Katz, eds, *Anti-Semitism in Times of Crisis* (New York, 1991; paperback edition, 1993).

4 ANXIETY IN THE AFRICAN AMERICAN AND BAME COMMUNITIES

1 Oliver Laughland and Lauren Zanolli, 'Why Is Coronavirus Taking Such a Deadly Toll on Black Americans? Longstanding Health and Socio-economic Disparities Have Made Minorities More Vulnerable to Covid-19', *The Guardian*, 25 April 2020, at www.theguardian.com.

2 Cary Funk and Alec Tyson, 'Intent to Get a COVID-19 Vaccine Rises to 60% as Confidence in Research and Development Process Increases', Pew Research Center, 3 December 2020, www.pewresearch.org.

3 K. Bailey, 'Structural Racism and Health Inequities in the USA: Evidence and Interventions', *The Lancet*, 389 (10077) (2017), pp. 1453–63; R. Nong, 'Patient-Reported Experiences of Discrimination in the U.S. Health Care System', *JAMA Network Open* 3 (2020), e2029650–e2029650; A. V. Dorn, R.E. Cooney, M. L. Sabin, 'COVID-19 Exacerbating Inequalities in the U.S.', *The Lancet*, 395 (2020) (10232), pp. 1243–4.

4 Jonathan Wosen and Andrea Lopez-Villafaña, 'We're Closer Than Ever to a COVID-19 Vaccine: That Has Some San Diegans of Color Concerned', *San Diego Union-Tribune*, 22 November 2020, at www.sandiegouniontribune.com.

5 Sharon Otterman, '"I Trust Science", Says Nurse Who Is First to Get Vaccine in U.S.', *New York Times*, 14 December 2020, at www.nytimes.com.

6 Cassi Pittman Claytor, *Black Privilege: Modern Middle-class Blacks with Credentials and Cash to Spend* (Palo Alto, CA, 2020).

7 Durand Jean-Yves and Cunha Manuela Ivone, '"To All the Anti-Vaxxers Out There…': Ethnography of the Public Controversy about Vaccination in the Time of COVID-19', *Social Anthropology*, 10 (18 May 2020), DOI: 10.1111/1469-8676.12805.

8 Charles M. Blow, 'How Black People Learned Not to Trust: Concerns About Vaccination Are Unfortunate, But They Have Historical Root', *New York Times*, 6 December 2020, at www.nytimes.com. This is a constant trope, as the Michele L. Norris writes a similar column three days later in the *Washington Post*, 'Black People Are Justifiably Wary of a Vaccine. Their Trust Must Be Earned', 9 December 2020, at www.washingtonpost.com. On the general background of these statements see Harriet A. Washington, *Medical Apartheid: The Dark History of Medical Experimentation on Black Americans from Colonial Times to the Present* (New York, 2006). Other recent studies of value in this context are Rana A. Hogarth, *Medicalizing Blackness: Making Racial Difference in the Atlantic World, 1780–1840* (Chapel Hill, NC, 2017) and Zinzi D. Bailey et al., 'Structural Racism and Health Inequities in the USA: Evidence and Interventions', *The Lancet*, 389 (2017), pp. 1453–63.

9 David McBride, *From TB to AIDS: Epidemics among Urban Blacks since 1900* (New York, 1991) and Cathy Cohen, *Boundaries of Blackness: AIDS and the Breakdown of Black Politics* (Chicago, IL, 1999).

10 Priscilla Wald, *Contagion: Cultures, Carriers, and the Outbreak Narrative* (Durham and London, 2008), p. 256 (Ebola); p. 234 (HIV/AIDS).

11 'In the Latest Sign of Covid-19-related Racism, Muslims Are Being Blamed for England's Coronavirus Outbreaks', *CNN Wire*, 6 August 2020, at www.cnn.com.

12 'Volunteers Needed: Would You Test a COVID-19 Vaccine for $1,100?' *Deseret Morning News*, 9 March 2020, at www.deseret.com.

13 'Boosting Diversity in COVID-19 Vaccine Clinical Trials', *Pharma and Healthcare Monitor Worldwide*, 3 December 2020, at https://hub.jhu.edu.

14 Fisher Jack, 'President Obama Tells Joe Madison He Will "Absolutely" Take Vaccine if Dr. Fauci Says It's Safe / LISTEN', *Newstex Blogs EUR/Electronic Urban Report*, 2 December 2020, at https://eurweb.com.

15 See Sasha Turner, 'Slavery and the Production, Circulation and Practice of Medicine', *Social History of Medicine*, XXXI/4 (November 2018), pp. 870–76; Rana A. Hogarth, *Medicalizing Blackness: Making Racial Difference in the Atlantic World, 1780–1840* (Chapel Hill, NC,

2017); Jim Downs, *Sick from Freedom: African-American Illness and Suffering During the Civil War and Reconstruction* (New York, 2012).

16 Joseph P. Williams, 'From Tuskegee to COVID: Diversity, Racism Are Hurdles in Drug Trials', USNEWS.com, 19 November 2020, at www.usnews.com.

17 Here we are echoing the work of Allan M. Brandt's path-breaking essay of 1978: 'Racism and Research: The Case of the Tuskegee Syphilis Study', *Hastings Center Report*, 8 (1978), pp. 21–9. This essay led eventually to the best-selling work of James H. Jones, *Bad Blood: The Tuskegee Syphilis Experiment* (New York, 1993), p. 17, which we shall discuss in much more detail below.

18 The reader will note that we have indicated where the various players were Jewish, as we believe strongly that their roles in both Black health and education were if not determined than impacted by their own sense of marginality. This was true for Julius Rosenwald at the beginning of the twentieth century as well as Peter Buxtun, who was a refugee during the Second World War.

19 See the work of Benjamin Roy, 'The Tuskegee Syphilis Experiment: Medical Ethics, Constitutionalism, and Property in the Body', *Harvard Journal of Minority Public Health*, 1 (1995), pp. 11–15, and 'The Julius Rosenwald Fund Syphilis Seroprevalence Studies', *Journal of the National Medical Association*, 88 (1996), pp. 315–22.

20 William D. Bryan, *The Price of Permanence: Nature and Business in the new South* (Athens, GA, 2018), p. 133ff for a detailed discussion of turn-of-the-century Black attitudes towards public health.

21 Alan M. Kraut, *Goldberger's War: The Life and Work of a Public Health Crusader* (New York, 2003).

22 See Sander L. Gilman, *Stand Up Straight! A History of Posture* (London, 2018), pp. 202ff.

23 See www.cdc.gov/tuskegee/timeline.htm, accessed 9 December 2020.

24 Alexandra Minna Stern, 'Eugenics Beyond Borders: Science and Medicalization in Mexico and the United States West, 1900–1950', dissertation, University of Chicago (1999); *Eugenic Nation: Faults and Frontiers of Better Breeding in Modern America* (Los Angeles and Berkeley, CA, 2005).

25 Jinbin Park, 'Historical Origins of the Tuskegee Experiment: The Dilemma of Public Health in the United States', *Uisahak: Korean Journal of Medical History*, 26 (2017), pp. 545–78.

26 Sander L. Gilman, 'Black Bodies, White Bodies: Toward an Iconography of Female Sexuality in Late Nineteenth-century Art,

Medicine and Literature', in *Race, Writing and Difference*, ed. Henry
Louis Gates Jr (Chicago, IL, 1986), pp. 223–61.

27 In this context see the two collected volumes: *'Andersartigkeit'
und Identität in menschlichen Gesellschaften: Die Verantwortung der
Wissenschaften*, ed. Volker Roelcke and Heinz Schott (Stuttgart,
2020) (Acta Historica Leopoldina. Bd. 73) and *Silence, Scapegoats,
Self-reflection: The Shadow of Nazi Medical Crimes on Medicine and
Bioethics*, ed. Volker Roelcke, Sascha Topp and Etienne Lepicard
(Göttingen, [2014]).

28 Theresa Benedek, '"Case Neisser": Experimental Design, the
Beginnings of Immunology, and Informed Consent', *Perspectives
in Biology and Medicine*, 57 (2014), pp. 249–67.

29 John D. Arras, 'The Jewish Chronic Disease Hospital Case', in *The
Oxford Textbook of Clinical Research Ethics*, ed. Ezekiel J. Emanuel
et al. (Oxford and New York, 2008), pp. 73–9. For the primary
materials see Hyman 251 N.Y.S.2d 818 (1964), revd 258 N.Y.S.2d 397
(1965); Jay Katz, *Experimentation with Human Beings* (New York,
1972), pp. 9–65.

30 James P. McCaffrey, 'Hospital Accused on Cancer Study', *New
York Times*, 21 January 1964, p. 31, at www.nytimes.com; 'State
Broadens Cancer Inquiry', *New York Times*, 22 January 1964, p. 38,
at www.nytimes.com; Alexander Burnham, 'Test on Cancer to
Need Consent', *New York Times*, 23 January 1964, p. 28, at https://
timesmachine.nytimes.com; John Osmandson, 'Many Scientific
Experts Condemn Ethics of Cancer Injection', *New York Times*,
26 January 1964, p. 70, at https://timesmachine.nytimes.com.

31 R. Katz et al., 'Awareness of the Tuskegee Syphilis Study and the U.S.
Presidential Apology and Their Influence on Minority Participation
in Biomedical Research', *American Journal of Public Health*, 98
(2008), pp. 1137–42.

32 Peter Novick, *The Holocaust in American Life* (Boston, MA, 1999).

33 The first edition was Jones, *Bad Blood* (New York, 1981); James H.
Jones and N.M.P. King, 'Bad Blood Thirty Years Later: A Q&A with
James H. Jones', *Journal of Law, Medicine and Ethics*, 40 (2012),
pp. 867–72.

34 See L. L. Wall, 'The Medical Ethics of Dr J. Marion Sims: A Fresh
Look at the Historical Record', *Journal of Medical Ethics*, 32 (2006),
pp. 346–50; Terri Kapsalis, *Public Privates: Performing Gynecology
from Both Ends of the Speculum* (Durham, NC, 1997); Deirdre Cooper
Owens, *Medical Bondage: Race, Gender, and the Origins of American
Gynecology* (Athens, GA, 2017).

35 Rebecca Skloot, *The Immortal Life of Henrietta Lacks* (New York, 2010). On the reception of this text Letitia V. Fowler, 'Learning from Stories of Experience: Using Narrative as Pedagogy to Understand Racial and Ethnic Experiences in Medicine', dissertation, Michigan State University (2015); Vincent Bruyere, 'The Lived Exemplarity of HeLa: A Matter of Lifedeath', *Mosaic*, XLVIII/4 (December 2015), pp. 123–36; Lindsay Morton, 'Evaluating the Effects of Epistemic Location in Advocatory Literary Journalism', *Journalism*, 17 (2016), pp. 244–59.

36 Laughland and Zanolli, 'Why Is Coronavirus Taking Such a Deadly Toll on Black Americans?'

37 Lola Fadulu, 'Amid History of Mistreatment, Doctors Struggle to Sell Black Americans on Coronavirus Vaccine', *Washington Post*, 7 December 2020, at www.washingtonpost.com.

38 Warren Vieth, 'Bush Salts His Summer with Eclectic Reading List', *Los Angeles Times*, 16 August 2005, at www.latimes.com.

39 Matthew Mosk, 'George W. Bush in 2005: "If We Wait for A Pandemic to Appear, It Will Be Too Late to Prepare": A Book about the 1918 Flu Pandemic Spurred the Government to Action', 5 April 2020, https://abcnews.go.com.

40 George Santayana, *The Life of Reason, or the Phases of Human Progress*, ed. Marianne Wokeck and Martin Coleman (Cambridge, 2011), p. 172.

41 Michael Gill and Nirmala Erevelles, 'The Absent Presence of Elsie Lacks: Hauntings at the Intersection of Race, Class, Gender, and Disability', *African American Review*, 50 (2017), pp. 123–37, here 123.

42 Candace Owens, *Blackout: How Black America Can Make Its Second Escape from the Democratic Plantation* (New York, 2020), p. 166 on COVID-19.

43 Elizabeth Dwoskin and Josh Dawsey, 'The Trump Administration Wants to Take Credit for a Covid Vaccine: Trump Supporters Are Undermining It', *Washington Post*, 24 December 2020, at www.washingtonpost.com.

44 Danielle Cinone, 'WILD WORDS Candace Owens AGAIN Pushes Anti-Covid Vaccine Conspiracy Theory After Calling Dr Fauci and Bill Gates "Pure Evil"', *The Sun*, 19 December 2020, www.thesun.co.uk.

45 Andrew Naughtie, '"I Love Diamond and Silk": Trump Stands by Controversial Sisters "Fired" by Fox Over Conspiracy Theories; Diamond and Silk Speculated that Coronavirus Is Man-made and that Death Count Is Being Inflated for Political Reasons', *The Independent*, 29 April 2020, at www.independent.co.uk.

46 Interview with NewsMax TV, 11 December 2020, at https://rumble.com.
47 Dickens Olewe, 'Stella Immanuel: The Doctor Behind Unproven
Coronavirus Cure Claim', BBC News, 29 July 2020, at www.bbc.com.
48 'Dino Melaye Makes Bogus, Unscientific Claims Against
COVID-19 Vaccine', Premium Times, 17 December 2020, at
www.premiumtimesng.com.
49 The complex role of self-identified Jews on the Right during the
pandemic, as we discussed in Chapter Three, put them in alliance
with radical antisemites that postulated a global Jewish conspiracy
as the cause of the pandemic as well as the force behind the
vaccination movement. Gold was in 2003 'marginally affiliated
to Judaism, [and] has since attended several classes and Shabbat
dinners sponsored by the Los Angeles Intercommunity Kollel
(LINK), a year-old organization based at the Westwood Kehilla
that puts on Shalom Time and adult classes, many of them for
beginners'. Julie Gruenbaum-Fax, 'Unaffiliated Find Connection in
LINK', Jewish Journal, 18 September 2003, at www.jewishjournal.com.
50 Will Sommer, 'Demon Sperm Doctors Group that Met with Pence Is
Now Pushing COVID Vaccine Fears', Daily Beast, 15 December 2020,
at www.thedailybeast.com.
51 Tony Kirby, 'Evidence Mounts on the Disproportionate Effect of
COVID-19 on Ethnic Minorities', The Lancet: Respiratory Medicine, 8
(8 May 2020), pp. 547–8, at www.thelancet.com.
52 Institute for Fiscal Studies (IFS), 'Are Some Ethnic Groups More
Vulnerable to COVID-19 Than Others?', 1 May 2020, at www.ifs.
org.uk.
53 Michael Drummond, 'Coronavirus-related Racism in Schools
Increasing, Union Warns Government', Regional Press Releases:
Wales (4 March 2020), at https://advance.lexis.com.
54 Sarwar Alam, '"BAME Communities Need to Take Extra Precautions,
to Ensure the Safety of the Most Vulnerable", Says Councillor Hina
Bokhari', Eastern Eye UK (23 March 2020), at www.easterneye.biz.
55 Baroness Doreen Lawrence, 'Summary', in An Avoidable Crisis: The
Disproportionate Impact of COVID-19 on Black, Asian and Minority
Ethnic Communities, 26 October 2020, at www.lawrencereview.
co.uk.
56 Baroness Doreen Lawrence, 'End Structural Racism', in An Avoidable
Crisis.
57 Smitha Mundasad, 'Ethnic Minority Covid Risk "Not Explained
by Racism"', BBC News, 22 October 2020, at www.bbc.com.
58 On medicine, status and marginality see Julian Simpson, Migrant

Architects of the NHS: South Asian Doctors and the Reinvention of British General Practice (1940s–1980s) (Manchester, 2019).

59 Elaine Robertson and Kelly S. Reeve et al., 'Predictors of COVID-19 Vaccine Hesitancy in the UK Household Longitudinal Study', *MedRxiv*, 2 January 2021, at www.medrxiv.org.

60 Christine Vestal, 'Health Care Workers Can Decline a COVID-19 Shot – For Now', *Pew Trust* (8 December 2020), at www.pewtrusts.org.

61 Royal College of Psychiatrists, *Impact of COVID-19 on Black, Asian, and Minority Ethnic (BAME) Staff in Mental Healthcare Settings, Assessment, and Management of Risk* (13 May 2020; updated 24 June 2020), at www.rcpsych.ac.uk.

62 Public Health England, *Disparities in the Risk and Outcomes of COVID-19* (August 2020), at https://assets.publishing.service. gov.uk.

63 Marie-Claude Gervais, 'The Drivers of Black and Asian People's Perceptions of Racial Discrimination by Public Services: A Qualitative Study', *ETHNOS Research and Consultancy, Department for Communities and Local Government* (January 2008), at https:// dera.ioe.ac.uk.

64 David Baddiel, *Jews Don't Count: How Identity Politics Failed One Particular Identity* (London, 2021), p. 52.

65 Ibid., p. 53.

66 On the background see Tudor Parfitt, *Hybrid Hate: Conflations of Antisemitism and Anti-Black Racism from the Renaissance to the Third Reich* (Oxford, 2020).

67 David Olusoga, 'Britain Is Not America. But We Too Are Disfigured by Deep and Pervasive Racism', *The Guardian*, 7 June 2020, at www.theguardian.com.

68 Nora Fakim and Cecilia Macaulay, '"Don't call me BAME": Why Some People Are Rejecting the Term', *BBC News*, 30 June 2020, at www.bbc.co.uk.

69 David van Heel and Vagheesh Narasimhan, 'Genetics and South Asian Populations', *Genes and Health*, at www.genesandhealth.org; Oliver Moody, 'Poor Health Among British Asians May Be in the Genes', *The Times*, 13 March 2015, at www.thetimes.co.uk.

70 Sandy Gupta, 'South Asian Background and Heart Health', *Heart Matters*, www.bhf.org.uk, accessed 10 December 2020.

71 Debate in the House of Lords in Response to the report by the All-Party Parliamentary Group on Obesity, *The Future of Obesity Services*, published on 25 November 2020, *Hansard*, 809 (5 January 2021), at https://hansard.parliament.uk.

72 On fat, ethnicity and race see Sander L. Gilman, *Fat: A Cultural History of Obesity* (Cambridge, 2008), pp. 101–23; 126ff.; *Obesity: The Biography* (Oxford, 2010), pp. 147ff.

73 Zahra Raisi-Estabragh et al., 'Greater Risk of Severe COVID-19 in Black, Asian and Minority Ethnic Populations Is Not Explained by Cardiometabolic, Socioeconomic or Behavioural Factors, or by 25(OH)-Vitamin D Status: Study of 1326 Cases from the UK Biobank', *Journal of Public Health*, XLII/3 (2020), pp. 451–60, https://academic. oup.com.

74 Rebecca Sheridan et al., 'Why Do Patients Take Part in Research? An Overview of Systematic Reviews of Psychosocial Barriers and Facilitators', *Trials*, 259 (12 March 2020), DOI: 10.1186/s13063-020-4197-3; https://trialsjournal.biomedcentral.com.

75 Mark Duell, 'Ethnic Minorities Are Significantly LESS Likely to Take the Coronavirus Vaccine Despite Being At Much GREATER Risk of the Disease, Says Study', *MailOnline*, 16 December 2020, at www.dailymail.co.uk.

76 Ibid.

77 Ali Ahmed et al., 'Outbreak of Vaccine-preventable Diseases in Muslim Majority Countries', *Journal of Infection and Public Health*, XI/2 (2018), pp. 153–5, at www.sciencedirect.com.

78 Ben Kasstan, 'Vaccines and Vitriol: An Anthropological Commentary on Vaccine Hesitancy, Decision-Making and Interventionism among Religious Minorities', *Anthropology and Medicine* online (2020), pp. 1–9, EBSCOhost, DOI: 10.1080/13648470.2020.1825618, as well as Paul A. Offit and Rita K. Jew, 'Addressing Parents' Concerns: Do Vaccines Contain Harmful Preservatives, Adjuvants, Additives, or Residuals?' *Pediatrics*, 112 (December 2003), pp. 1394–7, EBSCOhost, DOI: 10.1542/peds.112.6.1394.

79 Ben Kasstan, *Making Bodies Kosher: The Politics of Reproduction among Haredi Jews in England* (Oxford, 2019), pp. 231–2.

80 Ben Kasstan, '"A Free People, Controlled Only by God": Circulating and Converting Criticism of Vaccination in Jerusalem', *Culture, Medicine, Psychiatry*, 4 February 2021. DOI: 10.1007/s11013-020-09705-2.

81 'People Fearful of Taking Part in Vital Clinical Research', *Science News* (16 March 2020), at www.sciencedaily.com.

82 A. S. Forster et al., 'Ethnicity-specific Factors Influencing Childhood Immunisation Decisions among Black and Asian Minority Ethnic Groups in the UK: A Systematic Review of Qualitative Research', *Journal of Epidemiological Community Health*, 71 (2017), pp. 544–9, here 544, at https://jech.bmj.com.

83 Luke Haynes, 'GPS Demand Explanation Over BAME Omission from COVID Vaccine Priority List', GP Online, 7 December 2020, at www.gponline.com.

84 Mary Dejevsky, 'If Ethnic Minorities Are More Vulnerable to Covid, Should They Receive the Vaccine First?' The Independent, 4 December 2020, at www.independent.co.uk.

85 Nadine White, 'It's Harder for Black and Asian People to Trust the COVID Vaccine: Here's What Needs to Happen', Huffington Post UK, 11 December 2020, www.huffingtonpost.co.uk.

86 Vahé Nafilyan et al., "Ethnic Differences in COVID-19 Mortality During the First Two Waves of the Coronavirus Pandemic: a Nationwide Cohort Study of 29 Million Adults in England', medRxiv preprint, 5 February 2021, DOI: 10.1101/2021.02.03.21251004.

87 Hannah Recht and Lauren Weber, 'Black Americans Are Getting COVID Vaccines at Lower Rates Than White Americans', Scientific American, 20 January 2021, www.scientificamerican.com.

88 Abby Goodnough and Jan Hoffman, 'The Wealthy Are Getting More Vaccinations, Even in Poorer Neighborhoods', New York Times, 2 February 2021, at www.nytimes.com.

89 'Ethnic Minority Groups Less Likely to Take COVID Vaccine', Understanding Society (18 January 2021), at www.understandingsociety.ac.uk.

90 Press Ganey, 'Vaccine Hesitancy and Acceptance: Data Segmentation Helps Address Barriers' (20 January 2021), at http://images.healthcare.pressganey.com.

91 Ibid., p. 6.

92 'Every GP Practice Across Leicester, Leicestershire and Rutland Now Providing Covid-19 Vaccinations for Patients', NHS: Leicester City, at www.leicestercityccg.nhs.uk; Shanti Das, 'The Doctor Calls – to Persuade Covid Vaccine Refuseniks', The Times, 7 March 2021, at www.thetimes.co.uk.

5 TRUMP AS SYMBOL: ANGER WITHIN AND AGAINST 'WHITE' COMMUNITIES

1 This chapter deals with 'White' as a conceptual category. As we have already seen, ultra-Orthodox Jews and African Americans can be aligned with this perspective. What 'White' means here is the position that privileges the symbolic register of the existing established majority and relabels them as 'marginalized' or 'at risk'. See recently Neil Altman, White Privilege: A Psychoanalytic Perspective (New York, 2021). Here James David Dickson, 'Confidential FBI

Informant Details How He Infiltrated Group Accused in Whitmer
Kidnap Plot', *Detroit News*, 5 March 2021, at www.detroitnews.com.

2 David D. Kirkpatrick and Mike McIntire, "'Its Own Domestic Army':
How the G.O.P Allied Itself with Militants', *New York Times*,
8 February 2021, at www.nytimes.com.

3 Amy Brittain et al., 'The Capitol Mob: A Raging Collection of
Grievances and Disillusionment', *Washington Post*, 10 January 2021,
at www.washingtonpost.com.

4 Charlie Langton and Jay Dillon, 'Michigan Attorney Says "Burn Your
Masks" and Forget COVID Emergency Orders after State Supreme
Court Decision', *FOX2 Detroit*, 5 October 2020, at www.fox2detroit.
com.

5 Isaiah Berlin, 'Two Concepts of Liberty', in his *Liberty: Incorporating
'Four Essays on Liberty'*, ed. Henry Hardy (Oxford, 2002), pp. 166–
217. See also Isaiah Berlin, *The Idea of Freedom: Essays in Honor of
Isaiah Berlin*, ed. Alan Ryan (Oxford, 1979).

6 Thomas Hobbes, *Leviathan, or the Matter, Forme and Power of
a Commonwealth Ecclesiastical and Civil*, ed. Michael Oakeshott
(Oxford, 1960), p. 140.

7 Francesca Falk, *Eine gestische Geschichte der Grenze: Wie der Liberalismus
an der Grenze an seine Grenzen kommt* (Paderborn, 2011), pp. 63–90.

8 Hobbes, *Leviathan*, p. 114.

9 William Blackstone, *Blackstone's Commentaries on the Laws of England*
[1765–70], Book 4, chap. 13, at https://avalon.law.yale.edu. He further
defines 'the right of personal security' as consisting 'in a person's
legal and uninterrupted enjoyment of his life, his limbs, his body,
his health, and his reputation' (Book 1, chap. 1). And in his notes to
that same chapter he observes that 'For there is no man so indigent
or wretched, but he may demand a supply sufficient for all the
necessities of life from the more opulent part of the community.'

10 '. . . health and quarantine laws of the several States are not
repugnant to the Constitution of the United States, although
they affect foreign and domestic commerce, as in many cases
they necessarily must do in order to be efficacious, because until
Congress has acted under the authority conferred upon it by the
Constitution, such state health and quarantine laws producing
such effect on legitimate interstate commerce are not in conflict
with the Constitution.' *Compagnie Francaise de Navigation a Vapeur
v. Louisiana State Bd. of Health*, 186 U.S. 380, 387 (1902), at https://
biotech.law.lsu.edu/cases/pp/Compagnie.htm. See also *Asbell v.
Kansas*, 209 U.S. 251 (1908).

11 Matiangai Sirleaf, 'Responsibility for Epidemics', *Texas Law Review*, 97 (2018–19), pp. 285–354, at https://texaslawreview.org, as well as her 'COVID-19 and Allocating Responsibility for Pandemics', *JURIST – Academic Commentary*, 31 March 2020, at www.jurist.org.

12 Cass R. Sunstein and Adrian Vermeule, *Law and Leviathan: Redeeming the Administrative State* (Cambridge, MA, 2020), pp. 50–56, 58–61, 67–70, 76–7, 80–81, 84–5, 86–7, 125. We do understand the problems of adjudication and delegation as raised by Douglas H. Ginsburg and Steven Menashi, 'Nondelegation and the Unitary Executive', *University of Pennsylvania Journal of Constitutional Law*, XII/2 (2010), pp. 251–76. There can be, of course, gross misuse of such administrative powers, as we have seen regularly in the Trump administration. But where appropriate adjudication can take place without an ideological preconception, as in the anti-lockdown, anti-masking, anti-vaxxing ideologies of the far-right wing, such interventions are not only appropriate but necessary.

13 Ibid., p. 40.

14 Ibid., p. 5.

15 Luke Mogelson, 'The Militias Against Masks', *New Yorker* (17 August 2020), at www.newyorker.com.

16 Wesley Dockery, 'Who Are the Wolverine Watchmen? Members Involved in Michigan Kidnapping Plot Support QAnon "Deep State" Conspiracies', at *Newstex Blogs International Business Times News*, 9 October 2020, at www.ibtimes.com.

17 On 'post-truth' see Andrew Jewett, *Science Under Fire: Challenges to Scientific Authority in Modern America* (Cambridge, MA, 2020).

18 Brett Samuels, 'Trump Says Proud Boys Should "Stand Down" After Backlash to Debate Comments', *The Hill*, 30 September 2020, at https://thehill.com.

19 Elizabeth Dwoskin and Josh Dawsey, 'The Trump Administration Wants to Take Credit for a Covid Vaccine: Trump Supporters Are Undermining It', *Washington Post*, 24 December 2020, at www.washingtonpost.com.

20 'Donald Trump Speech "Save America" Rally Transcript January 6', *Transcript Library*, 6 January 2021, at www.rev.com.

21 Carlton F. W. Larson, ''Shouting "Fire" in a Theater': The Life and Times of Constitutional Law's Most Enduring Analogy', *William and Mary Bill of Rights Journal*, 24 (2015–16), pp. 181–212, at https://scholarship.law.wm.edu.

22 Mick Brown, 'Is There Any Truth Behind the Covid-19 Conspiracy Theories?; Was Covid-19 Created in a Lab, Spread by 5G Masts,

Or Does It All Come Back to Bill Gates? Inside the Insidious World of Conspiracy Theories', *The Telegraph*, 27 June 2020, at www.telegraph.co.uk.

23 Glenn Kessler, 'Trump Is Averaging more than 50 False or Misleading Claims a Day', *Washington Post*, 22 October 2020, at www.washingtonpost.com.

24 Glenn Kessler, 'Trump Made 30,573 False Or Misleading Claims as President: Nearly Half Came in His Final Year', *Washington Post*, 23 January 2021, at www.washingtonpost.com.

25 All citations are to Miles T. Armaly and Adam M. Enders, "Why Me?" The Role of Perceived Victimhood in American Politics', *Political Behavior*, 43 (in press, 20 January 2021), DOI: 10.1007/s11109-020-09662-x.

26 'Remarks by President Trump on Infrastructure, Charlottesville Rally', *Newstex Blogs Voice of America*, 15 August 2017, at www.voanews.com.

27 Claudia Schmölders, *Hitler's Face: The Biography of an Image* (Philadelphia, PA, 2006), pp. 34ff, and Sander L. Gilman and Claudia Schmölders, eds, *Gesichter der Weimarer Republik: eine physiognomische Kulturgeschichte* (Cologne, 2000).

28 Gavriel D. Rosenfeld, 'An American Fuehrer? Nazi Analogies and the Struggle to Explain Donald Trump', *Central European History*, 52 (2019), pp. 554–87; Jeffrey Herf, 'Lessons from German History after Charlottesville', *History News Network* (HNN), 9 October 2017, at https://historynewsnetwork.org (this article focuses on differences between Nazi Germany in 1933 and the United States in 2017. It also addresses the term 'anti-fascism' that has returned as the much-maligned 'antifa'. Herf concludes with a look at German efforts to come to terms with the Nazi past after 1945 as compared to the engagement of the American South with the Civil War); Christopher Browning, 'The Suffocation of Democracy', *New York Review of Books* (25 October 2018), at www.nybooks.com (this article connects the American present to the late Weimar era, comparing Mitch McConnell damage to democracy with that wrought by Hitler's conservative allies who helped him into power); Helmut Walser Smith, 'No, America Is Not Succumbing to Fascism', *Washington Post*, 1 September 2020, at www.washingtonpost.com (this article points to the differences between Nazi Germany and the United States and ultimately rejects the analogy); Alberto Toscano, 'The Long Shadow of Racial Fascism', *Boston Review*, 28 October 2020, at www.bostonreview.net (the author seeks to 'dislodge the debate

about fascism from the deadlock of analogy' by turning to the long history of Black radical thinking. He points out that 'For people of color at various historical moments, the experience of racialization within a liberal democracy could have the valence of fascism'); Benjamin Carter Hett, 'What the Bunker Mentality Really Means', *Los Angeles Times*, 15 November 2020, at www.latimes.com.

29 [Interview with historian Richard Evans], 'Democracy Dies in a Variety of Ways', *Slate*, 12 July 2018, at https://slate.com.

30 Cyndee Miller, 'Even Without HIV Issue, Using Celebs Can Be Risky', *Marketing News TM*, 9 December 1991, at https://advance.lexis.com.

31 Lawrence Donegan and Paul Webster, 'Focus: Fast-food Slump: Mctrouble: Times Are Lean for the Company that Has Come to Symbolise American Corporate Might, Report Lawrence Donegan in San Francisco and Paul Webster in Paris', *The Observer*, 20 October 2002, at www.theguardian.com.

32 'World Highlights for Wednesday December 30', *AAP Newsfeed*, 30 December 2020, at https://advance.lexis.com.

33 Harold D. Lasswell, *Politics: Who gets What, When, How* (New York, 1939), p. 87.

34 Cited by Lee Grieveson, *Cinema and the Wealth of Nations Media, Capital, and the Liberal World System* (Berkeley, CA, 2017), p. 387.

35 Edward Bernays, *Propaganda* (New York, 1928), p. 9.

36 Cathy Gelbin and Sander L. Gilman, *Cosmopolitanisms and the Jews* (Ann Arbor, MI, 2017), pp. 145ff.

37 Kristian Blickle, 'Pandemics Change Cities: Municipal Spending and Voter Extremism in Germany, 1918–1933', *Federal Reserve Bank of New York Staff Reports*, no. 921 (May 2020), at www.newyorkfed.org.

38 Nico Voigtländer and Hans-Joachim Voth, '(Re)-shaping Hatred: Anti-Semitic Attitudes in Germany, 1890–2006', *CEPR Discussion Paper 8935* (London, 2012).

39 [Review of] *Der ewige Jude* [The Eternal Jew], *Unser Wille und Weg*, 10 (1940), pp. 54–5.

40 Stephen Braun, Hope Yen and Calvin Woodward, 'AP FACT CHECK: Trump and the Virus-era China Ban that Isn't', *Associated Press*, 18 July 2020, at www.apnews.com.

41 Josh Boak and Christopher Rugaber, 'AP FACT CHECK: Trump Says Economy Best "EVER." It's Not', *Associated Press*, 4 June 2018, at www.apnews.com.

42 Jonathan Jarry, 'The Anti-vaccine Movement in 2020', *McGill: Office of Science and Society*, 22 May 2020, at www.mcgill.ca.

43 Abby Phillip, Lena H. Sun and Lenny Bernstein, 'Vaccine Skeptic Robert Kennedy Jr. Says Trump Asked Him to Lead Commission on "Vaccine Safety"', *Washington Post*, 10 January 2017, at www.washingtonpost.com.

44 Bob Weber, 'Provinces Seen as Unable to Protect Ecology', *Globe and Mail* (Canada), 18 September 2003, at www.theglobeandmail.com.

45 Michael Hiltzik, 'Trump Attacks Biden and Harris as Anti-vaccine, But He's the One with the Anti-vaxx Record', *Los Angeles Times*, 8 September 2020, at www.latimes.com.

46 Washington Post Staff, 'Wednesday's GOP Debate Transcript, Annotated', *Washington Post*, 16 September 2015, at www.washingtonpost.com.

47 Marc A. Thiessen, 'The Ten Best Things Trump Did in 2020', *Washington Post*, 31 December 2020, at www.washingtonpost.com.

48 At https://childrenshealthdefense.org, accessed 23 December 2020.

49 At www.facebook.com/rfkjr/posts/2826857840974280, accessed 23 December 2020.

50 Evan Halper and Chris Megerian, 'THE NATION: Biden Gets Vaccine as Trump Hedges; Many Wondering Why White House Ceding Spotlight on a Rollout Seen as Huge Triumph', *Los Angeles Times*, 22 December 2020, at www.latimes.com.

51 Kerry Kennedy Meltzer, 'Vaccines Are Safe, No Matter What Bobby Kennedy Says', *New York Times*, 30 December 2020, at www.nytimes.com.

52 'Beck: Anti-vaxxers Are Being Persecuted, Just Like Galileo', US *Official News*, 4 February 2015, at https://advance.lexis.com.

53 Maggie Haberman, 'Trump and His Wife Received Coronavirus Vaccine Before Leaving the White House', *New York Times*, 1 March 2021, at www.nytimes.com.

54 Sam Dorman, 'Trump Takes Credit for "China Virus" Vaccine: "I hope everyone remembers"!' *Fox News*, 10 March 2021, at www.foxnews.com.

55 Celine Castronuovo, '49 Percent of GOP Men Say They Won't Get Vaccinated: PBS Poll', *The Hill*, 11 March 2021, at www.thehill.com.

56 Stephen Robinson, '2020: The Year Trump's Dummies Wouldn't Wear Masks', *Newstex Blogs Wonkette*, 1 January 2021, at https://advance.lexis.com

57 Reuters Staff, 'Herman Cain, Ex-Presidential Candidate Who Refused to Wear Mask, Dies After COVID-19 Diagnosis', *Reuters*, 30 July 2020, at www.reuters.com.

58 Christina Pazzanesse, 'Calculating Possible Fallout of Trump's Dismissal of Face Masks', *Harvard Gazette*, 27 October 2020, at https://news.harvard.edu.

59 Michael D. Shear et al., '"Covid, Covid, Covid": In Trump's Final Chapter, a Failure to Rise to the Moment', *New York Times*, 31 December 2020, at www.nytimes.com.

60 Ashley Collman, '2 Days Before His Coronavirus Diagnosis, Trump Mocked Biden for Wearing a Face Mask', *Business Insider*, 2 October 2020, at www.businessinsider.com. Bob Woodward's *Rage* appeared with Simon & Schuster in New York on 15 September 2020. It contained detailed discussions about the then president's knowledge and obfuscations based on transcriptions of their conversations beginning in February 2020 and centring on the pandemic: see chapters 30 (pp. 212ff.); 32 (242ff.), 36 (275ff.), 37 (284ff.), 38 (299 ff); 41 (333ff.), 43 (349ff.), 44 (352ff.), 46 (379ff.).

61 Ryan Suppe, 'Amid Stay-home Order, Ammon Bundy Hosts Meeting; Calls on Idahoans to Defend Rights', *Idaho Press*, 27 March 2020, at www.idahopress.com.

62 Anna Maria Barry-Jester et al, 'Pandemic Backlash Jeopardizes Public Health Powers, Leaders', *Kaiser Health News*, 15 December 2020, at www.khn.org.

63 Ivan Pereira, 'Ammon Bundy Arrested 2nd Straight Day for Violating Idaho Statehouse Ban', *ABC News*, 26 August 2020, at https://abcnews.go.com.

64 Christopher Mathias, 'Ammon Bundy Leads Protest at Home of Idaho Cop Who Arrested Anti-vaxxer', *Huffington Post*, 23 April 2020, at www.huffpost.com.

65 Brittany Bernstein, 'Ammon Bundy Comes Out in Support of BLM, Calls to Defund the Police, *National Review*, 31 July 2020, at www.nationalreview.com.

66 Michael M. Grynbaum, Davey Alba and Reid J. Epstein, 'How Pro-Trump Forces Pushed a Lie about Antifa at the Capitol Riot', *New York Times*, 1 March 2021, at www.nytimes.com.

67 Zechariah Chafee Jr, 'Freedom of Speech in War Time', *Harvard Law Review*, XXXII/8 (1919), pp. 932–73.

68 M. Tyler Gillett, 'Justice Alito Gives Speech Criticizing Decisions Regarding Religious Freedom', *Jurist*, 14 November 2020, at www.jurist.org.

69 All quotes are from www.supremecourt.gov/search.aspx?filename=/docket/docketfiles/html/public/20a90.html, accessed 23 December 2020.

70 All quotes are from www.supremecourt.gov/opinions/20pdf/
20a136_bq7c.pdf, accessed 8 February 2021.

71 Luis Pérez-González, '"Is Climate Science taking over the Science?":
A Corpus-based Study of Competing Stances in *Bias*, *Dogma*
and *Expertise* in the Blogosphere', *Humanities and Social Sciences
Communication*, vii/92 (15 September 2020), at www.nature.com.

72 Philip Oltermann, 'Ginger Root and Meteorite Dust: The Steiner
"Covid Cures" Offered in Germany', *The Guardian*, 10 January 2021,
at www.theguardian.com.

73 Rachel Leishman, 'QAnon Disappointed to Find jfk Jr. is, in Fact,
Dead – Not Trump's New Running Mate', *Newstex Blogs: The Mary
Sue*, 19 October 2020, at https://advance.lexis.com.

74 Blackstone, *Blackstone's Commentaries on the Laws of England*, Book 1,
chap. 1.

75 Mark Mackinnon and Nathan Vanderlippe, 'How the Coronavirus
Pandemic Is Making Strongmen Stronger, from Hungary to Serbia
to the Philippines', *The Globe and Mail*, 6 April 2020, at www.
theglobeandmail.com.

76 Königlichen Preußischen Akademie der Wissenschaften, ed., *Kants
gesammelte Schriften* (Berlin, 1900–), iv, pp. 402. See also Andrews
Reath, 'Legislating the Moral Law', *Nöus*, 28 (1994), pp. 435–64, and
John Rawls, 'Kantian Constructivism in Moral Theory', *Journal of
Philosophy*, 77 (1980), pp. 515–72, reprinted in his *Collected Papers*
(Cambridge, ma, 1999), pp. 303–58.

77 Sigmund Freud, *The Standard Edition of the Complete Psychological
Works of Sigmund Freud*, ed. James Strachey, vol. xxi (1927–31): *The
Future of an Illusion, Civilization and its Discontents, and Other Works*
(London, 1953), p. 103.

6 MARGINALITY AND DISEASE

1 Charles E. Rosenberg, 'The Definition and Control of Disease –
An Introduction', *Social Research*, 55 (1988), pp. 327–30, here 327.
Rosenberg was clearly using hiv/aids to show the illusionary claim
of modern medicine that, by the end of the 1970s, it had conquered
infectious disease. hiv/aids was a painful reminder that medicine
was far from triumphant, as it claimed. As with hiv/aids, covid-19
today is another reminder that modern medicine is far from having
conquered infectious disease. Yet the successful vaccine rollout in
some wealthy Western countries as well as the resulting gradual
'opening up' and hence the demand for a return to 'normality', at

least for some, would allow many quickly to forget the widespread dread of the pandemic. This was certainly the case in sections of the United States in the spring of 2021.

2 See Sander L. Gilman and J. M. Thomas, *Are Racists Crazy? How Prejudice, Racism, and Antisemitism Became Markers of Insanity* (New York, 2016), pp. 132ff.

3 David Rieff, *In Praise of Forgetting: Historical Memory and its Ironies* (New Haven, CT, 2016), p. 4.

4 See in this context Caroline Hovanec, 'Of Bodies, Families, and Communities: Refiguring the 1918 Influenza Pandemic', *Literature and Medicine*, 29 (2011), pp. 161–81.

5 Elizabeth Outka, *Viral Modernism: The Influenza Pandemic and Interwar Literature* (New York, 2019), p. 244.

6 Ibid., p. 255.

7 Tom Dicke, 'Waiting for the Flu: Cognitive Inertia and the Spanish Influenza Pandemic of 1918–19', *Journal of the History of Medicine and Allied Sciences*, 70 (2015), pp. 195–217, here 197.

8 In general, see John Fabian Witt, *American Contagions: Epidemics and the Law from Smallpox to Covid-19* (New Haven, CT, 2020).

9 J. Leeds Barroll III, *Politics, Plague, and Shakespeare's Theater: The Stuart Years* (Ithaca, NY, 1991), pp. 156ff. See also Stephen Greenblatt, 'What Shakespeare Actually Wrote About the Plague', *New Yorker*, 7 May 2020, at www.newyorker.com.

10 For example, Vanessa Thorpe, 'A Happy Ending for King Lear? Trauma of Plague Caused Shakespeare to Change Play's Finale', *The Observer* (London), 13 December 2020, at www.theguardian. com; Gregory Doran, 'How Shakespeare's Work Was Shaped by a Covid-like Crisis', *The Times* (London), 15 December 2020, at www.thetimes.co.uk.

11 Daniel Reid, 'Epidemic', in *The Oxford Companion to the Body*, ed. Colin Blakemore and Sheila Jannett (Oxford, 2003), pp. 249–50, here p. 249.

12 Thomas Lodge, *A treatise of the plague containing the nature, signes, and accidents of the same, with the certaine and absolute cure of the feuers, botches and carbuncles that raigne in these times: and aboue all things most singular experiments and preseruatiues in the same, gathered by the obseruation of diuers worthy trauailers, and selected out of the writing of the best learned phisitians in this age* (London, 1603), p. 45v.

13 Gideon Harvey, *Morbus anglicus: or, The anatomy of consumptions Containing the nature, causes, subject, progress, change, signes, prognosticks, preservatives; and several methods of curing all*

consumptions, coughs, and spitting of blood. With remarkable observations touching the same diseases. To which are added, some brief discourses of melancholy, madness, and distraction occasioned by love. Together with certain new remarques touching the scurvy and ulcers of the lungs (London, 1666), p. 3.

14 John Milton, *The Divorce Tracts of John Milton: Texts and Contexts, 1608–1674*, ed. Sara J. van den Berg and W. Scott Howard (Pittsburgh, PA, 2010), p. 166.

15 See Mark Honigsbaum, *The Pandemic Century: One Hundred Years of Panic, Hysteria, and Hubris* (New York, 2020), updated edition of the 2019 study with an epilogue on COVID-19; Tera L. Martin, 'Epidemic Time: AIDS and the Imagining of American Cultural History', dissertation, University of California, Santa Cruz (2000).

16 Reuters Staff, 'H1N1 Flu Must Be Global Before Phase 6 – WHO Chief', 21 May 2009, at www.reuters.com.

17 'WHO Director-General's Opening Remarks At the Media Briefing on COVID-19', 11 March 2020', at www.who.int.

18 Richard E. Neustadt and Ernest R. May, *Thinking in Time: The Uses of History for Decision Makers* (New York, 1986).

19 *Swine Flu Immunization Program: Supplemental Hearings Before the House Committee on Interstate and Foreign Commerce. Subcommittee on Health and the Environment . . . Ninety-fourth Congress* (Washington, DC, 1976), p. 442.

20 Glenn Kessler, 'In Context: What Biden Aide Ron Klain Said About the Swine Flu', *Washington Post*, 15 October 2020, at www.washingtonpost.com.

21 Zhou Xun, 'Postcard: Countdown to Chaos in Beijing', *Far Eastern Economic Review*, 15 May 2003, p. 49; Robert F. Breiman et al., 'Role of China in the Quest to Define and Control SARS', in *Learning from SARS: Preparing for the Next Disease Outbreak*, ed. Knobler et al. (Washington, DC, 2004), pp. 56–62.

22 Elaine Showalter, *Hystories: Hysterical Epidemics and Modern Culture* (London, 1997).

23 Stephen L. Muzzatti, 'Bits of Falling Sky and Global Pandemics: Moral Panic and Severe Acute Respiratory Syndrome (SARS)', *Illness, Crisis and Loss*, 13 (2005), pp. 117–28.

24 Private communication, 23 April 2003. See Zhou Xun, 'Postcard', p. 49.

25 Private communication, 21 April 2003.

26 Jock Young, 'The Role of the Police as Amplifiers of Deviance, Negotiators of Drug Control as Seen in Notting Hill', in *Images of Deviance*, ed. Stanley Cohen (Harmondsworth, 1971), pp. 27–61.

27 Sandy Sufian and Licia Carlson, 'Thoughts on Precarity, Disablement, and Risk during COVID-19', in *Defining the Boundaries of Disability: Critical Perspectives*, ed. Licia Carlson and Matthew C. Murray (New York, 2021), pp. 124–37, here pp. 125–6.

28 Craig Swan, 'SPL Star's Swine Flu Terror as His Little Girl Stops Breathing; Killie Ace's Fears for Tot Hayden', *Daily Record*, 28 November 2009, at www.dailyrecord.co.uk.

29 Alison Phillips, '"I Was Terrified Thinking about What Could Have Happened to my Jake . . . "; Exclusive: Coleen's Swine Flu Agony', *The Mirror*, 10 July 2009.

30 'Local Teens Describe their Experiences with Swine Flu', *Washington Post*, 25 August 2009, at www.washingtonpost.com.

31 Sufian and Carlson, 'Thoughts on Precarity, Disablement, and Risk during COVID-19', p. 125.

32 Sara Ahmed, *The Cultural Politics of Emotion* (Edinburgh, 2004) as well as Laura Otis, *Banned Emotions: How Metaphors Can Shape What People Feel* (New York, 2019).

FURTHER READING

Barry, John M., *The Great Influenza: The Story of the Deadliest Plague in History* (New York, 2005)

Davis, Mark, and Davina Lohm, *Pandemics, Publics, and Narrative* (Oxford, 2020)

Diamond, Jared, *Guns, Germs, and Steel: The Fates of Human Society* (New York, 1997).

Douglas, Mary, *Purity and Danger: An Analysis of Concepts of Pollution and Taboo* (New York, 1966).

Evans, Richard J., *Death in Hamburg: Society and Politics in the Cholera Years, 1830–1910* (Oxford, 1987)

Gilman, Sander L., *Disease and Representation: Images of Illness from Madness to AIDS* (Ithaca, NY, 1988)

Hays, J. N., *Epidemics and Pandemics: Their Impacts on Human History* (Santa Barbara, CA, 2005)

Hogarth, Rana A., *Medicalizing Blackness: Making Racial Difference in the Atlantic World, 1780–1840* (Chapel Hill, NC, 2017)

Honigsbaum, Mark, *The Pandemic Century: One Hundred Years of Panic, Hysteria, and Hubris* (New York, 2020)

Huremović, Damir, ed., *Psychiatry of Pandemics: A Mental Health Response to Infection Outbreak* (Cham, 2019)

Kraut, Allan, *Silent Travelers: Germs, Genes, and the 'Immigrant Menace'* (New York, 1994)

McMillen, Christian W., *Pandemics: A Very Short Introduction* (Oxford, 2016)

McNeill, William H., *Plagues and Peoples* (Garden City, NY, 1976)

Makari, George, *Of Fear and Strangers: A History of Xenophobia* (New York, 2021)

Markel, Howard, *Quarantine!: East European Jewish Immigrants and the New York City Epidemics of 1892* (Baltimore, MD, 1999)

Napier, David, *The Age of Immunology: Conceiving a Future in an Alienating World* (Chicago, IL, 2003)

Rosenberg, Charles E., *Explaining Epidemics* (Cambridge, 1992)
Snowden, Frank M., *Epidemics and Society: From the Black Death to the Present* (New Haven, CT, 2019)
Washington, Harriet A., *Medical Apartheid: The Dark History of Medical Experimentation on Black Americans from Colonial Times to the Present* (New York, 2006)
Watts, Sheldon J., *Epidemics and History: Disease, Power, and Imperialism* (New Haven, CT, 1997)
Zhou Xun, *The People's Health: Health Intervention and Delivery in Mao's China, 1949–1983* (Montreal, 2020)